HEALTH AND HEALTH CARE UTILIZATION IN LATER LIFE

Edited by

Jon Hendricks

Oregon State University

Perspectives on Aging and Human Development Series
Jon Hendricks: Series Editor

BAYWOOD PUBLISHING COMPANY, INC.

Amityville, New York

Library of Congress Catalog Number: 94-20403
ISBN: 0-89503-168-X

Library of Congress Cataloging-in-Publication Data

Health and health care utilization in later life / edited by Jon
  Hendricks.
      p.   cm. - - (Perspectives on aging and human development
series)
    Includes bibliographical references (p.   ).
    ISBN 0-89503-168-X
    1. Aged- -Health and hygiene- -Social aspects.   2. Aged- -Social
conditions.   3. Aged- -Mental health- -Social aspects.   4. Aged-
-Social networks.   5. Aged- -Medical care. I. Hendricks, Jon, 1943-
. II. Series.
RA564.8.H397 1995
362.1'9897- -dc20   94-20403
                                                              CIP

Table of Contents

Introduction
THE PICTURE OF HEALTH:
BRINGING HUMAN BEINGS BACK IN

Jon Hendricks

WHAT PRICE WELL-BEING?

There is no shortage of questions about the nature of health. Almost everyplace one looks these days it is possible to find some kind of discussion about one or another aspect of health, health care delivery and utilization. One common theme that quickly emerges is that what we know is dwarfed by what we do not know. It seems the questions proliferate while the answers are maddingly elusive.

Health and health care utilization are among those topics about which most of us have an opinion. With the election of President Clinton, the politics of health care, long simmering on the back burner, was suddenly moved to the front and the temperature turned up. It could well be that other industrialized countries will reconsider their policies but for now the United States is the sole industrialized country in the world without national health insurance. Even so, we spend a greater percentage of our Gross Domestic Product on health care than most of our neighbors. Having said that, it must also be said that for any argument made on any side of the issue, there is undoubtedly a counter argument. One thing is sure, however, the status of health care in the United States is not an anomaly insofar as the underlying moral economy of the country is concerned. In a recent volume edited by Navarro [1], many of the contributors assert that health care is no different than the provision of many other human services—it is hinged to our basic beliefs in a market economy and the proprietarization of essential services. Interest group politics rule the day, the question for us is: Who speaks for the elderly?

Best-guess forecasts, to borrow a phrase Wolfe [2] recently used to introduce *The Coming Health Crisis,* are bleak. Interest groups have aligned themselves on one or the other side of the current debate over national health insurance and the "disinformation" campaigns are in full-swing. What has not been fully explicated in the media blitz is that the thirty-six million of us without health insurance have done little or nothing to make the quandary in which we find ourselves. The same goes for the elderly. The fact that the oldest-old, the most rapidly growing segment of the population, exert a disproportionate draw on the nation's health resources is, in part, a result of the very successes in which the country takes so much pride. Of course we all ought to have enough sense to engage in preventative nutrition, smoking cessation programs, low stress occupations, bucolic life styles, but with an exercise regime, and everything else that will improve our health profiles. But look around, which way are the advertising tides running? Is Dave out there pitching healthy life styles or fast food? Is the tobacco lobby promoting alternative crops or subsidies? As one looks at one's peers or one's mirrors, it is not difficult to see where the battle of the bulge is being won.

Yet, we persist in pointing fingers at those who seek medical care and seem to assume they are responsible for their own condition. Bad as that tendency is, it gets even worse when we cast funding for whatever attention they might require as a form of intergenerational transfer. The nomenclature is left over from the expansionist phase of the country's history. The ideology, however, is beginning to reflect a pattern of competing demands during a time of economic contraction. The next generation is not going to be larger than those going through the lifecourse already. In fact, if we carefully examine the so-called "pig in the python" phenomena, it is clear that the python better start looking elsewhere [2]. It is a different kind of mistake to think that poor health or inadequate access is just a problem for those who are old or those who have to go without. It is a problem for all of us. Binstock and Post [3] phrased the same debate in terms of the question, *Too Old for Health Care?* As a nation are we ready to impose any form of rationing on the health care so commonly thought to be a basic right of citizenship? During the 1980s any number of "trial balloons" were lofted: the funny thing about "trial balloons" is that they do not have to soar in order to begin to change the way people think.

BROADENING THE PERSPECTIVE

Moving beyond the debate about the delivery and funding of health care, the issues are just as obstinate. Much as we would like it to be the case, no realm of human functioning is insulated from any other realm of functioning. Anyone who has ever blushed or had any other type of physical response to an external stimuli that had some particular emotional significance will realize on a visceral level that mind and body are not all that distinct. We may like to think of them as different but that do not function independently.

There is a range of social and behavioral factors that have a direct impact on definitions of health and health functioning. The first two subsections to follow address a few of these factors. From the concern with the role of gender in health, to the plight of the elderly, the social construction of health goes on unabated [4]. The subordination of any number of critical issues of aging health concerns is a case in point. As yet, we have a very narrow perspective on what constitutes the health picture for people as they age.

The chapters in this collection are intended to expand our horizons on this question a bit. As the major subsections imply, health is concatenated from a combination of physical and mental health, from contextual and definitional factors, and from the social networks in which individuals find themselves. In itself that claim is not particularly earth shattering. It is not until one stops to think that the typical health care provider is schooled in a single aspect or that even when a team or health maintenance approach is taken an integrated perspective is difficult to obtain. Then too, primary prevention is seldom a priority for health care providers faced with waiting rooms full of people seeking immediate relief for existing conditions.

All too frequently, physical and mental health are seen as distinct not only from one another, but from other aspects of an older person's life. Physical and mental health interact in inexorable ways. The conditions a person has and that person's frame of mind are embedded in the context of their life worlds and the types of services available to them. To understand how each of these dimensions operates, we need to understand how they interact with one another. As Davis-Berman contends, sense of self-efficacy is crucial on both sides of the question. Impaired functioning in one realm is going to challenge one's sense of efficacy and have consequences in the other realm. While consensus is sometimes ephemeral, the belief that social support has a salutatory effect for physical and mental health comes pretty close to achieving universal affirmation in health research. That is not to say that social support networks are not themselves stressful, they certainly can be [5]. Nonetheless, the absence of support for a person who would benefit from being nurtured can be devastating.

If it were not so serious, the extent of the myths about physical and mental health for urban and rural elderly would be amusing. It is assumed, far too frequently, that the advantages on either score all accrue to those who reside in urban areas—the mythology of the bucolic lifestyle aside. In three of the chapters to follow this distinction is roundly challenged. That is not to say that rural disadvantages are non-existent, only to claim, as do Stolar, MacEntee and Hill, that context is crucial.

Part of what constitutes context are the ascribed variables that people carry with them as they navigate the lifecourse. Ory and Warner [4], along with many other researchers, have helped emphasize that such things as gender are not just another variable to be considered. As long as gender is seen as a dummy variable, male or not-male, it is unlikely that significant research results will be forthcoming.

Being female is hardly the same thing as being not-male. Nelson attempts to specify how race and gender interact with social support to affect the way health service utilization occurs.

Having read the chapters in this volume readers will surely find themselves with more questions than answers. That is as it should be.

REFERENCES

1. V. Navarro (ed.), *Why the United States Does Not Have a National Health Program,* Baywood, Amityville, New York, 1993.
2. J. R. Wolfe, *The Coming Health Crises: Who Will Pay for the Care of the Aged in the Twenty-first Century?* University of Chicago Press, Chicago, 1993.
3. R. H. Binstock, and S. G. Post (eds.), *Too Old For Health Care?* Johns Hopkins University Press, Baltimore, 1991.
4. M. Ory and H. R. Warner (eds.), *Gender, Health and Longevity: Multidisciplinary Perspectives,* Springer, New York, 1990.
5. J. R. Johnson, *Factors Associated with Negative Actions between Caregivers and Care-Receivers,* presented to the annual meeting of the Gerontological Society of America, 1993.

Section I

Physical and Mental Health in the Later Years

Chapter 1

LIFE EVENTS, SOCIAL SUPPORT, AND IMMUNE RESPONSE IN ELDERLY INDIVIDUALS

William Alex McIntosh, Howard B. Kaplan, Karen S. Kubena, and Wendall A. Landmann

There is ample and growing evidence that implicates psychosocial factors in immune response both in vivo and in vitro [1]. Little consensus exists, however, regarding relevant parameters and on the particular factors such as age or gender that moderate this relationship [1].

Few studies, for instance, have focused on elderly individuals. Because of naturally declining immunocompetence, elderly individuals may be less prone to stress-induced immunologic change. However, Kennedy, et al. argue that, because elderly individuals have weaker immune systems, psychosocial distress may *increase* the risk of illness [2]. In addition, as elderly individuals frequently follow restricted diets and take a number of medications, both of which affect immunocompetence, studies that account for dietary adequacy, nutritional status, and the use of medications are needed.

Similarly, few studies have sought to differentiate the psychosocial factors that affect men's and women's immune systems. While gender (as well as age) is usually used as a statistical control in studies of the psychological-immune response relationship, some studies have focused directly on gender differences in immune system function [3]. One explanation of the observed differential points to hormonal factors [4], while another, to stress differences associated with the social identity of gender [1].

A study of nutritional factors in elderly individuals provided the opportunity to address some of these issues, although the original intent of the research was not to focus on the immune system. The present research focuses on the relationship between stressful life events and immunocompetence in a sample of free-living elderly men and women. This relationship is examined, taking into account social support, psychological adjustment, the use of lymphocyte-altering medications, nutritional status, and socio-demographic background. Since support, adjustment, the effect of life events, and immune functioning vary with gender, particular attention is paid to this factor.

Kaplan's Psychosocial Model of Immunosuppression

Kaplan developed a model of immunosuppression that groups social and psychological factors that affect immunocompetence into four categories: dysphoric responses or psychological adjustment, immunosuppressive behaviors, adverse life experiences, and vulnerability (see Figure 1) [1].

Dysphoric Responses

A number of studies implicate the experience of dysphoria with lower immune response, where dysphoria is represented by unhappiness, anxiety, or depression. Linn, et al. found that "t-lymphocytic" response was reduced in bereaved individuals who were rated as depressed [5]. Women with severe symptoms of depression were more likely to have impaired killer cell activity [6]. Others have found either higher white blood cell counts or lower killer cell activity in individuals with high scores on indicators of anxiety [7-9].

Adverse Life Experiences

It has long been thought that negative changes in the individual's circumstances increase the risk of illness [10]. One form of adverse circumstance involves often abrupt, acute life changes such as losing one's job, having one's spouse die, or having one's home burglarized. Researchers have implicated the appearance of such "life events" with lower immune functioning [11-13]. When stressful life event scales were used, elevated immunogloblin levels were found among rheumatoid arthritis patients with increased life change scores [14]. First year medical students with high stressful life event scores had lower levels of natural killer cell activity [15], and women with high levels of life change were found to have lower killer cell activity [16]. Other specific stressful events such as participation in manned spaceflights, fellowship examinations, and divorce/ separation also have been reported to lower immunocompetence [12, 13, 17-20].

Other, more chronic conditions may serve as adverse life experiences. These include role strain as reflected in marital conflict, the pressures associated with holding multiple roles, and low social evaluation of certain roles. Men who experience conflict with their spouses were more likely to experience greater distress and lower helper-suppressor ratios [21]. Multiple role responsibilities were associated with greater distress and lower percentage of t-lymphocytes and

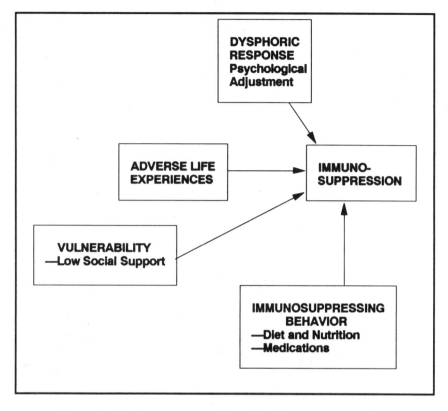

Figure 1. Kaplan's psychosocial model of immunosuppression.

helper t-lymphocytes among caregivers of family members with Alzheimer's disease than in a comparison group [12].

Immunosuppressive Behaviors

A number of behaviors such as sleep patterns, alcohol consumption, tobacco use, drug use, and diet affect immune response as well. Lack of sleep reduced t-cell count and increased white blood cell count [21] as did protein calorie malnutrition [22] and diets deficient in vitamins, minerals, and amino acids [23-24].

Vulnerability

Immune response is lower in the presence of vulnerability or the inability to cope with adverse life events. Coping includes personal dispositions such as hardiness [25] or ego-strength [26]. Social relationships also constitute a means of coping. Social support was positively associated with a lower risk of mortality from chronic illness [27] and depression [28]. The presence of social support buffered or protected the individual from such consequences by providing companionship, comfort, and the sense that others care. The absence of social support increased the effects of adverse life experiences [29].

Kaplan suggests a complex model of immunosuppression involving the direct effects of the four psychosocial factors as well as their interrelations [1]. The model makes no claims regarding the relative effects of these four factors on immunosuppression, but does suggest that low levels of social support do not directly reduce immune response, but rather lead to immunosuppression by increasing the impact of adverse life experiences and dysphoric response. Other literature suggests that high levels of social support reduce dysphoric response and the impact of adverse life circumstances. Since some research has found evidence of social support as either a mediating or buffering factor in stress-health conditions, these additional effects need to be considered.

Age and Gender

The literature concerning the four categories of psychological and social factors involved in immunocompetence tends to focus on non-elderly individuals. The relevance of these findings for elderly individuals remains unclear. It is arguable that since elderly individuals experience health problems, stressful circumstances [31], and social support [32] that differ from younger individuals, new psychosocial models of immune response may be needed for elderly individuals.

The research discussed above not only lacks insights regarding elderly individuals but also pays little attention to gender. Men and women experience health differently and this differential experience holds true in old age. Men die more quickly while women experience greater illness [33]. Men and women encounter different life events [34], and more universal life circumstances have a differential impact on one gender versus the other [32, 35]. For example, men with low levels of social support are more vulnerable to illness and mortality than women. In view of these considerations, the interrelationships among the four psychosocial factors and immunosuppression will be examined by gender.

Since the need for psychosocial studies of immune response that focus on elderly persons and that examine the differential experience of males and females is apparent, this study seeks to:

1. determine which psychosocial factors predict immune response in elderly males and in elderly females, controlling for relevant factors; and,
2. compare the direct, mediating, and buffering effects of social support in these models.

METHODOLOGY

The data utilized in this study are drawn from the "Social Support, Stress, and the Aged's Diet and Nutrition" project. The sample consists of 424 elderly Houstonians (age 58 or more) randomly selected from two sources. The first source was random digit dialing; 355 of the respondents were located in this way. Random sampling from the membership lists of American Association of Retired Persons (AARP) and selected churches constitute the second source.[1] The sample draws respondents from the Houston SMSA (Texas) which includes a six county area. Blood samples were tested for immune response.[2]

The blood samples were maintained at a temperature below 4C and shipped in styrofoam mailing packs with extra padding by bus to the laboratory in College Station for analysis. Upon receipt in College Station, the serum was transformed to a labeled vial and stored at −30 Celsius (C). The heparinized blood was centrifuged (IEC Central-7 Model Centra, International Equipment Company, Needham Heights, Massachusetts) at 400 × g for fifteen minutes. The EDTA tubes were taken for analysis at St. Joseph's Hospital Laboratory, Bryan, Texas in 192 cases.[3]

Dependent Variable

Immunocompetence is measured by total lymphocyte count (TLC) (number/ mm^3), using a Coulter Counter Model S-Plus V to assay samples. The number of lymphocytes varies over a twenty-four-hour period. Blood samples were taken at various times during the day. Consequently, diurnal variation in number of

---

[1] Despite the differences in sampling frames, the elderly from both groups are highly similar in terms of health, socioeconomic status, and even participation in voluntary organizations.

[2] Three 7-ml tubes of blood were drawn from each person by a trained phlebotomist. One tube contained ethylenediamine tetraacetic acid (EDTA) as an anticoagulant (Vacutainer, Bectin-Dickinson, Rutherford, New Jersey) and was used for plasma separation. The second tube (evacuated serum separation tube, Vacutainer, Bectin-Dickinson) was centrifuged (Centrific model 228, Fisher Scientific, Fair Lawn, New Jersey) at 400 × g for thirty minutes to separate the serum for the remaining blood components. The third tube contained heparin. Because interviews took place at varying times of the day, it was not possible to obtain fasting blood samples.

The blood samples were maintained at a temperature below 4C and shipped in styrofoam mailing packs with extra padding by bus to the laboratory in College Station for analysis. Upon receipt in College Station, the serum was transferred to a labeled vial and stored at −30 Celsius (C). The heparinized blood was centrifuged (IEC Central-7 Model Centra, International Equipment Company, Needham Heights, Massachusetts) at 400 × g for fifteen minutes. The EDTA tubes were taken for analysis at St. Joseph's Hospital Laboratory, Bryan, Texas.

[3] An attempt was made to draw a blood sample from all individuals. However, the phlebotomists were instructed to cease in their attempts if a vein either could not be easily located or it collapsed during the attempted draw. Forty-seven blood samples were not drawn as a result. In addition, transportation and storage of the blood samples led to varying degrees of hemolysis (red cell breakdown) in an additional 188 samples.

lymphocytes could have affected results. This was not taken into account in the analysis.

Control and Independent Variables

Nutritional Status

Albumin served as a non-nutrient specific, global indicator of nutritional status. Albumin in serum was determined colorimetrically at 628 nm on a Beckman DB spectrophotometer with Sigma Diagnostic Kit, Procedure No. 631-2 (Sigma Diagnostic, St. Louis, Missouri). This is based upon the ability of the protein to bind bromcresol green to form a measurable chromagen [36]. Expected values were 3.2-4.0 g/dl.

Lymphocyte Affecting Drugs

Certain medications either elevate or suppress lymphocyte count [37]. Respondents were asked to indicate whether they currently were taking medications of any sort. Those who took medications were asked to produce their containers so that an accurate recording of the medication name and its recommended dosage could be made. A dummy variable was formed, with those elderly individuals currently taking lymphocyte-reducing medication coded as "1" ($n = 47$) and those not taking such medication coded as "0." None of the respondents from whom blood was drawn were taking lymphocyte-elevating drugs.

Recent Life Events

Life events are defined as occurrences of disruptions which result in stress because of the "failure of routine methods for managing threats" [38]. We utilized a shortened version of the Holmes and Rahe life-event scale which focuses on life events particularly relevant to elderly individuals [39]. The twenty-three-item scale was adapted from Blazer and Mensh [40, 41]. Since men and women experience life events differentially and the occurrence of these events have a differential impact by gender, we *did* not form summary scales. Instead, we treated each life event separately, and examined whether the occurrence, recency, longevity, and disruptiveness of each event affects immune response [42]. In addition, each event was coded with regard to the simultaneous occurrence of 1) having occurred within one month prior to the interview and 2) having been rated by the respondent as very upsetting.

Psychological Adjustment

A series of items, drawn from Nagi, indicating the degree to which the respondent had difficulties with sleep, nervousness or anxiety, rapid heartbeat, fainting spells, or shortness of breath was used to reflect psychological adjustment [43]. A principal components analysis produced a single factor that explained 65 percent of the variation in these items and produced a theta reliability coefficient of 0.54.

Social Support

Indicators of social support follow closely those of Claude Fischer and Eugene Litwak [44, 45]. The respondents were asked to indicate whether they received any of seventeen kinds of help (with everyday living needs such as cooking, companionship, comfort, home repairs, loans of money or household items, advice about food, finances, or government programs, etc.). The names of all those individuals providing such help were obtained.

We used these lists of names to generate information about the respondents' intimate networks. After Fischer, the five names (or less) that appeared most frequently were identified as the respondents' intimate networks [44]. A series of questions about each of the five individuals was asked to determine the composition (percent kin, percent friends, percent former coworkers, etc.) of the intimate network. In addition, the respondents were asked how frequently they got together with each member of their intimate network (1 = almost never; 3 = very frequently). A frequency of interaction score was then formed for each respondent based on the average frequency for getting together with intimates.

FINDINGS

Initially, a series of t-tests determined whether the variables in the model (i.e., immune response, psychological distress, life events) varied by gender. As expected, elderly females reported significantly higher levels of psychological maladjustment than elderly males. For many life events, no significant difference in occurrence, duration, recency, or amount of disruption appeared by gender. However, elderly females were more likely to report the occurrence, and greater recency, duration, and impact of minor physical illness, minor financial difficulties, losing one's driver's license, having a concern for the physical well-being of a family member, relationship problems with other family members, and legal problems. Elderly men experienced more sexual problems than females and reported more recent occurrence as well as the more negative impact of such problems. No differences by gender in either lymphocyte count (males $\bar{x} = 217.96$ number/mm^3, $s.d. = 143.00$; females $\bar{x} = 230.25$ number/mm^3; $s.d. = 128.63$) or albumin (males $\bar{x} = 4.37$ g/dl, $s.d. = 0.68$; females $\bar{x} = 4.45$ g/dl, $s.d. = 0.61$) were observed.

Regression analyses were run separately for the male and female samples. Percent kin, as the only social support variable to correlate significantly with lymphocyte count, was selected to appear in the model for males. For similar reasons, recency of sexual problems and length of a family member's illness were the only two life event variables selected for the model. Examination of column 1 in Table 1 reveals that, of the two, only recency of sexual problems has a significant effect ($p < .05$) on lymphocyte count—thus the more recent a sexual problem for males, the poorer their immune response. The addition of psychological adjustment to the equation (column 2) improves the fit; those males who

Table 1. Lymphocyte Count Regressed on Life Events, Background Characteristics, Nutritional Status, and Lymphocyte Affecting Drugs; Plus Psychological Adjustment; Plus Social Support (Males)

	β (1)	Beta	β (2)	Beta	β (3)	Beta
Recency of sexual problems	-15.442**	-.296	15.918**	-.305	-12.898*	-.247
Length of family illness	-8.188*	-.223	-7.582	-.206	-4.795	-.130
Psychological adjustment			4.614**	.336	50.230***	.321
Percent kin					129.944**	.270
Age	-2.583	-.104	-3.238	-.130	-3.153	-.126
Income	-2.710	-.035	-1.946	-.025	-.461	-.006
Education	4.5287	.116	3.633	.093	4.286	.110
Nutritional status	-8.417	-.0043	14.053	.071	3.273	.118
Lymphocyte reducing drugs	59.614	.154	68.649	.178	65.071	.169
Adjusted R^2	.032*		.113*		.168**	

*$p < 0.10$
**$p < 0.05$
***$p < 0.01$

experience psychological adjustment have a greater immune response. Finally, the equation in the third column includes percent kin in the intimate network—the higher the percentage of kin, the higher the immune response.

As the results in Table 2 indicate, very different effects are found for females. Only recent, disruptive stress from familial or legal problems are associated with lymphocyte count. However, the relationship is positive rather than inverse. Psychological adjustment has no effect on lymphocyte count. However, the hypothesized positive affect of interaction with intimates on the lymphocyte count was observed.

We next examined the various sorts of effects hypothesized for social support: direct, mediating, buffering after Wheaton [46]. From Table 1, for males, percent kin in the intimate network has a demonstrable direct effect. To test for a mediating effect, we calculated the direct effect that percent kin has operating through the stressful events. The magnitude (.05) of this effect is sufficiently small to argue that social support does not mediate stress. Similarly, it does not mediate psychological maladjustment. Finally, to test for buffering, interaction terms were formed between percent kin and the two life events, after trichotomizing percent kin into 0 = less than 1 *s.d.* below the mean; 1 = ± 1 *s.d.* above or below the mean; 2 = greater than 1 *s.d.* above the mean. Addition of these interactions to the original regression equations increased insignificantly the variance explained and

Table 2. Lymphocyte Count Regressed on Life Events, Background Characteristics, Nutritional Status, and Lymphocyte Affecting Drugs; Plus Psychological Adjustment (Females)

	β (1)	Beta	β (2)	Beta	β (3)	Beta
Recent, disruptive stress from familial and legal problems	120.909**	.209	124.749**	.215	127.017**	.221
Psychological adjustment			7.521	.057	6.848	.051
Interaction with intimates					49.245**	.258
Age	6.608***	.307	6.480**	.288	5.156**	.238
Income	7.371	.147	8.169	.156	6.438	.128
Education	−.657	−.018	−.577	−.016	−.865	−.024
Nutritional status	39.105*	.192	41.028*	.194	50.028*	.239
Lymphocyte affecting drugs	.680	.002	−1.152	−.090	6.069	−.018
Adjusted R^2	.088**		.087**		.125**	

*$p < 0.10$
**$p < 0.05$
***$p < 0.01$

neither term was statistically significant. Similarly, no buffering or mediating effects were detected in the model for females. We thus conclude that social support has a direct effect on immune response for males and females, but has neither mediating nor buffering effects.

DISCUSSION

Using Kaplan's psychosocial model of immune response, we sought to determine whether the same factors affecting immune response in younger populations affect elderly men and women in the same way [1]. We also investigated the role of social support (as a direct, mediating, or buffering factor) in this model. What we found indicates that the psychosocial model works well for elderly men and women. We also found that differing aspects of social support, have a direct positive impact on immune response for elderly males and females, but have no mediating or buffering effects.

Turning to the effects of psychological adjustment on immune response, the hypothesis holds for males but not for females. Among elderly males, the higher the psychological adjustment, the higher the lymphocyte count. However, psychological adjustment is not affected by recent experience of sexual dysfunction. Nor do males exhibit greater psychological adjustment with greater social support. In contrast, higher levels of adjustment have no such effect on elderly females.

The male-specific findings are striking in a number of respects. Most noteworthy of these, only recent sexual dysfunction affects immune function in multivariate analysis. Apparently, consistent with a review of literature on sexual dysfunction and its impacts on men and women, such dysfunction affects males more than it does females. While studies reveal that females in general are more likely to experience dysfunction, men suffer more from its psychological consequences [47, 48]. The greater impact on men may be accounted for by differential sex role expectations. Men may be subject to higher expectations regarding sexual performance. They are expected to take the initiative and have the potential to perform on demand. This responsibility requires an immediate, but sustained erection. The lack of such can not only lead to self-doubt and self-derogation, but spousal conflict as well [49]. Thus, while women generally report greater rates of sexual dysfunction, males more likely argue that it harms their marriages and are more likely to seek help for it [47]. Men's rates of sexual difficulties increase dramatically after age 65, while their sexual interest and activity remain high [49, 50].

The absence of any other significant stressful events may reflect the protected nature of the male participants' environment. These individuals are no longer part of the labor force. Many work-related stressors are not present. Sexual functioning may have thus increased in meaningfulness for these individuals, rendering sexual dysfunction highly problematic.

For elderly females, life events have little impact on psychological adjustment and, indeed, recent appearances of stress in family and legal areas have a *positive* effect on immune response. The differentials in roles and role responsibilities between men and women noted by others begin to lessen in old age [51-54]. Both have likely retired and children have grown up and left home. The social isolation previously experienced by women is lessened now that husbands are home. Women no longer face the pressures of balancing work and household responsibilities, and perhaps spouses more willingly participate in household maintenance. However, this peace may be achieved with a certain cost. Perhaps the very lessening of role differentials and responsibilities bring with it a lessening of challenges and feelings of worth [55]. The appearance of problems that impact the family offer renewed opportunities for meaningful involvement. Thus, "problems" have a positive effect on lymphocyte count.

The gender-specific correlates of lymphocyte count permit two interpretations. First, specific indicators of immune function may have different meanings for different segments of the population such as males and females. Others have argued in this regard that certain indicators may signify immunocompetence in some circumstances and immunosuppression in others [1]. Alternatively, for females as well as males, lymphocyte count may be indicative of immunocompetence, but for females the perception of stress in legal and familial areas may represent challenges, particularly for elderly females, that give meaning to life. In any case, these results suggest the continued need to examine the moderating effects of personal character on the relationship between stress and immune functioning as well as the need to consider a wide range of markers of immunocompetence and the benign or malignant significance of each of these for the functioning of the immune system. These results suggest that the stressful implications of life circumstances, individually or cumulatively considered, must take into account their differential affective significance for different segments of the population.

REFERENCES

1. H. B. Kaplan, Social Psychology of the Immune System: A Conceptual Framework and Review of Literature, *Social Science Medicine 33,* pp. 909-923, 1991.
2. S. Kennedy, J. C. Kiecolt-Glaser, and R. Glaser, Social Support, Stress, and the Immune System, in *Social Support: An Interactional View,* B. R. Sarason, I. G. Sarason, G. R. Pierce (eds.), John Wiley & Sons, New York, 1990.
3. H. C. Hendrie, F. Paraskevas, and J. Varsamis, Gama Globulin Levels in Psychiatric Patients, *Canada Psychiatric Association, 17,* pp. 93-97, 1972.
4. L. M. Verbrugge, Women and Men: Mortality of Older People, in *Aging in Society, Selected Reviews of Recent Research,* M. W. Riley, B. B. Hess, B. Bond (eds.), Lawrence Erlbaum Associates, Hillsdale, pp. 139-174, 1983.
5. M. W. Linn, B. S. Linn, and J. Jensen, Stressful Events, Dysphoric Mood, and Immune Responsiveness, *Psychological Reports, 54,* pp. 219-222, 1984.
6. M. Irwin, M. Daniels, E. T. Bloom, T. L. Smith, and H. Weiner, Life Events, Depressive Symptoms, and Immune Function, *American Journal of Psychiatry, 14,* pp. 437-441, 1987.
7. L. Temoshok, Psychoimmunology and AIDS, in *Psychological Neuropsychiatric, and Substance Abuse Aspects of AIDS,* Vol. 44, T. P. Bridge, A. F. Mirsky, and F. K. Goodwin (eds.), Raven Press, New York, pp. 187-197, 1988.
8. S. M. Levy, Behavioral Risk Factors and Host Vulnerability, in *Psychological Neuropsychiatric, and Substance Abuse Aspects of AIDS,* Vol. 44, T. P. Bridge, A. E. Mirsky, and F. K. Goodwin (eds.), Raven Press, New York, pp. 225-239, 1988.
9. S. E. Locke, M. W. Hurst, J. S. Heisel, L. Kraus, and R. M. Williams, The Influence of Stress on Immune Response, Annual Meeting of the American Psychosomatic Society, Washington, D.C., 1979.
10. B. S. Dohrenwend and B. P. Dohrenwend, Life Stress and Illness: Formulation of the Issues, in *Stressful Life Events and Their Contexts,* B. S. Dohrenwend and B. P. Dohrenwend (eds.), Rutgers University Press, New Brunswick, pp. 1-27, 1981.
11. J. K. Kiecolt-Glaser, R. Glaser, E. C. Shuttleworth, C. S. Dyer, P. Ogrocki, and C. E. Speicher, Chronic Stress and Immunity in Family Caregivers of Alzheimer's Disease Views, *Psychological Medicine, 49,* pp. 523-535, 1987.

12. S. J. Schleifer, S. E. Keller, M. Caerino, J. C. Thorton, and M. Stein, Suppressiosn of Lymphocyte Stimulation Following Bereavement, *Journal of the American Medical Association, 250,* pp. 374-377, 1983.
13. R. Glaser, J. K. Kiecolt, J. C. Stout, K. L. Tarr, C. E. Speicher, and J. E. Holliday, Stress-related Impairments in Cellular Immunity, *Psychiatric Research, 16,* pp. 223-239, 1985.
14. H. C. Hendrie, F. Paraskwas, F. P. Barager, and J. D. Adamoon, Stress, Immunoglobin Levels, and Early Polyarthritis, *J. Psychosomatic Research, 15,* pp. 337-342, 1971.
15. J. K. Kiecolt-Glaser, W. Garner, C. E. Speicher, G. M. Penn, J. Holliday, and R. Glaser, Psychosocial Modifiers of Immunocompetence in Medical Students, *Psychosomatic Medicine, 46,* pp. 7-14, 1984.
16. M. Irwin, M. Daniels, E. T. Bloom, T. L. Smith, and H. Weiner, Life Events, Depressive Symptoms, and Immune Function, *American Journal of Psychiatry, 14,* pp. 437-441, 1987.
17. S. L. Kimzey, P. C. Johnson, S. E. Ritzman, and C. E. Megel, Hematology and Immunology Studies: The Second Named Skylab Mission, *Aviation Space Environmental Medicine, 47,* pp. 383-390, 1976.
18. B. Dorian, P. E. Garfinkel, G. Brown, A. Shore, D. Gladman, and E. Keystone, Aberrations in Lymphocyte Subpopulations and Function during Psychological Stress, *Clinical Experimental Immunology, 50,* pp. 132-139, 1982.
19. R. W. Bartrop, E. Luckhurst, L. Lazarus, L. G. Kiloah, and R. Penny, Depressed Lymphocyte Function after Bereavement, *Lancet, 1,* pp. 834-836, 1977.
20. J. K. Kiecolt-Glaser, L. D. Fisher, P. Ogrocki, J. C. Scott, C. E. Speicher, and R. Glaser, Marital Quality, Marital Disruption, and Immune Function, *Psychosomatic Medicine, 49,* pp. 13-34, 1988.
21. J. Palmblad, Stress and Immunologic Competence: Studies in Man, in *Psychoneuro-Immunology,* A. Ader (ed.), Academic Press, Orlando, pp. 229-257, 1981.
22. B. R. Bistrian, G. L. Blackburn, and N. S. Scrimshaw, Cellular Immunity in Semistarved States in Hospitalized Adults, *American Journal of Clinical Nutrition, R8,* pp. 1148-1155, 1975.
23. J. Eskola, O. Raushamen, and E. Soppi, Effect of Sport Stress in Lymphocyte Transformation and Antibody Formation, *Clinical Experimental Immunology, 32,* pp. 339-345, 1978.
24. R. K. Chandra, Numerical and Functional Deficiency in T Helper Cells in Protein Energy Malnutrition, *Clinical Experimental Immunology, 51,* pp. 126-132, 1983.
25. S. C. Kobasa, Stressful Life Events, Personality, and Health: An Inquiry into Hardiness, *Journal Personality Social Psychology, 37,* pp. 1-11, 1979.
26. A. Canter, L. E. Cluff, and J. B. Imboden, Hypersensitive Reactions to Immunization, Innoculations, Antecedent Psychological Vulnerability, *Journal Psychosomatic Research, 16,* pp. 99-101, 1972.
27. L. F. Berkman, The Changing and Heterogeneous Nature of Aging and Longevity: A Social and Biomedical Perspective, in *Annual Review of Gerontology and Geriatics,* Vol. 8, G. L. Maddox and M. P. Lawton (eds.), Springer, New York, pp. 37-68, 1988.
28. W. M. Ensel and N. Lin, The Life Stress Paradigm and Psychological Distress, *Journal Health Social Behavior, 32,* pp. 321-341, 1991.

29. J. S. House, K. S. Landis, and D. Umberson, Social Relationships and Health, *Science, 241,* pp. 540-545, 1988.
30. K. G. Manton, Mortality and Morbidity, in *Handbook of Aging and the Social Sciences* (3rd. Edition), R. H. Binstock and L. K. George (eds.), Academic Press, San Diego, pp. 64-90, 1990.
31. J. S. House and C. Robbins, Age, Psychological Stress, and Health, in *Aging in Society: Selected Reviews of Recent Research,* M. W. Riley, B. B. Hess, and K. Bond (eds.), Lawrence Erlbaum Associates, Hillsdale, pp. 175-193, 1983.
32. T. C. Antonucci, Social Supports and Social Relationships, in *Handbook of Aging and the Social Sciences* (3rd. Edition), R. N. Binstock and L. K. George (eds.), Academic Press, San Diego, pp. 205-226, 1990.
33. L. M. Verbrugge, The Twain Shall Meet: Empirical Explanations of Sex Differences in Health and Mortality, *Journal Health Social Behavior, 30,* pp. 228-304, 1989.
34. L. I. Pearlin, The Sociological Study of Stress, *Journal Health Social Behavior, 30,* pp. 241-268, 1989.
35. M. Masuda and T. H. Holmes, Life Events: Perceptions and Frequencies, in *Life Change, Life Events, and Illness,* T. H. Holmes and E. M. David (eds.), Praeger, New York, pp. 289-318, 1989.
36. R. Corcoran and S. Duran, Albumin Determination by a Modified Bromcresol Green Method, *Clinical Chemistry, 23,* pp. 765-766, 1977.
37. Drug Interactions and Site Effects Index, Physician's Desk Reference (43rd Edition), Medical Economics Co., Inc., Oradell, 1982.
38. E. Gross, Organization, and Stress, in *Social Stress,* S. Irvine and N. P. Scotch (eds.), Aldine Press, Chicago, pp. 54-110, 1970.
39. T. H. Holmes and R. H. Rahe, The Social Readjustment Rating Scale, *Journal Psychosomatic Research, 11,* pp. 213-218, 1967.
40. D. Blazer, Social Support and Mortality in an Elderly Community Population, *American Journal Epidemiology, 115,* pp. 684-694, 1981.
41. I. N. Mensh, A Study of a Stress Questionnaire: The Later Years, *International Social Aging Human Development, 16,* pp. 201-207, 1983.
42. S. Henderson, D. C. Byrne, and P. D. Jones, *Neurosis and the Social Environment,* Academic Press, Sydney, 1981.
43. S. Z. Nagi, An Epidemiology of Disability among Adults in the United States, *Milbank Memorial Quarterly,* pp. 439-467, Fall 1976.
44. C. Fischer, *To Dwell among Friends: Personal Networks in Town and Country,* University of Chicago Press, Chicago, 1982.
45. E. Litwak, *Helping the Elderly: The Complementary Roles of Informal Networks and Formal Systems,* Guiliford Press, New York, 1985.
46. B. Wheaton, Models of the Stress-buffering Functions of Coping Resources, *Journal Health Social Behavior, 26,* pp. 352-364, 1985.
47. H. C. Helman and J. Verhulst, Gender and Sexual Functioning, in *Gender and Psychopathology,* I. Al-Issa (ed.), Academic Press, New York, pp. 305-320, 1982.
48. W. E. Stock, Sex Roles and Sexual Dysfunction, in *Sex Roles and Psychopathology,* C. S. Widom (ed.), Plenum Press, New York, pp. 249-275, 1984.
49. W. H. Masters and V. E. Johnson, *Human Sexual Response,* Little, Brown and Co., Boston, 1970.

50. L. E. Troll and B. F. Turner, Sex Differences in Problems of Aging, in *Gender and Disordered Behavior: Sex Differences in Psychopathology,* E. S. Sombey and V. Franks (eds.), Brunner/Mazel, New York, pp. 124-156, 1979.
51. S. Gore and T. W. Mangione, Social Roles, Sex Roles, and Psychological Distress: Additive and Interactive Models of Sex Differences, *Journal Health Social Behavior, 24,* pp. 300-312, 1983.
52. D. B. Kandel, M. Davies, and V. H. Ravers, The Stressfulness of Daily Social Roles for Women: Marital, Occupational and Household Roles, *Journal Health Social Behavior, 26,* pp. 64-78, 1985.
53. P. A. Thoits, Gender and Marital Status Differences in Control and Distress: Common Stress versus Unique Explanations, *Journal Health Social Behavior, 28,* pp. 7-22, 1987.
54. D. Belle, The Stress of Caring, Women as Providers of Social Support, in *Handbook of Stress: Theoretical and Clinical Aspects,* L. Goldberger and S. Breznitz (eds.), Free Press, New York, pp. 496-505, 1982.
55. J. Mirowsky and C. E. Ross, *Social Causes of Psychological Distress,* Aldine de Gruyter, New York, 1989.

Chapter 2

ASSOCIATIONS AMONG HEALTHY HABITS, AGE, GENDER, AND EDUCATION IN A SAMPLE OF RETIREES

J. Paul Leigh
and
James F. Fries

Healthy and unhealthy habits may be as or more important than access to medical care as variables that predict morbidity and monality. Cigarette use, lack of exercise, excessive alcohol use, lack of fiber, and excess fat in the diet have been linked to every major chronic disease [1, 2] and seat belt use has been linked to automobile crash deaths—the most frequent death-producing injury [3]. Yet, despite the research attention toward linking habits to disease and injury, little, by is research was supported in párt by a grant from the National Institutes of Health (AM21393) to ARAMIS (American Rheumatism Association Medical Information System). comparison, has been directed toward the correlates of the habits themselves. This is unfortunate. If policy variables, such as the level of education in the population, can be linked to habits, and if causality can be assumed to run from education to habits, then national efforts to raise education and awareness levels can be viewed as preventive medicine. The first purpose of this exploratory study is to investigate the association between education and habits. Since the data are derived from observation, as are virtually all large samples of people, causality cannot be demonstrated. But correlations can suggest where experimental studies and theory construction might be most useful. It is not always possible to demonstrate causal relations with data on human behavior. Within social science, for example, randomized trials have never been conducted to prove that a college education will increase a person's IQ. A literature search did not uncover any studies which investigated education and habits in a senior sample.

The second purpose is to test the hypothesis that healthy habits tend to be positively correlated with each other and negatively correlated with unhealthy habits. Evidence for these correlations are abundant and are attributed to individuals' desires for a healthy life [4-7]. An alternative theory is that healthy habits might be inversely related to each other since persons who are addicted to cigarettes or are alcoholics may compensate by exercising or eating foods high in fiber and low in fat [8, 9]. A final "null hypothesis" theory would suggest that the habits are independent of each other [10]. The "desire for a healthy life" versus the "compensating" or "null hypothesis" theories have yet to be tested in a sample consisting only of retirees.

The third purpose pertains to the specific habits themselves. Attempts will be made to determine which habits are most strongly correlated with other habits. For example, the frequent claim that excessive drinkers also tend to be excessive smokers will be investigated. Whether persons who have high fiber diets also eat less fat will be considered. Finally, we will consider which habit is most strongly associated with all of the others.

The fourth purpose is simply to assess the correlations between habits on the one hand and gender and age on the other. In samples including a wide age range: 1) Age is found to positively correlate with, for example, seat belt use [11] and; 2) Women are more likely than men to use seat belts [12].

Again, age, gender, and habits associations among retirees have not been widely investigated in the literature.

DATA AND METHODS

In 1986, Blue Shield contracted with Healthtrac, a health promotion firm in Palo Alto, California, to assess the health habits and health status of Bank of America retirees then residing in California. Healthtrac mailed questionnaires and follow-up newsletters and reminders to the 3,876 randomly selected retirees. One-thousand eight-hundred sixty-four retirees (1,864) returned these questionnaires in the initial survey. The sample may not be representative of all Bank of America retirees or retirees in general. It is likely, but cannot be directly documented, that respondents have slightly better health habits than non-respondents due to selection bias. But there are rebuttals to this non-random sample criticism. First, the sample is large—1,864 people. Second, information on six health habits is available—most prior studies considered only one or two. Third, this is an exploratory study which will generate hypotheses. We will not claim that results here would necessarily be transferred to retirees in general.

While Healthtrac collected information six months and twelve months later, during March, 1988 and November, 1988 the data in this study are drawn from the initial survey from November, 1987 so that attrition bias will not be present. Information was gathered pertaining to age, gender, years of schooling, together with a wide range of health habits.

Means and univariate correlation coefficients are calculated, and multiple regressions are run using SAS software [13].

Results

Table 1 presents definitions, means, and standard deviations of the variables used in the analysis. Some of the variables in Table 1 deserve special attention. "Fiber" indicates the number of times each week the respondent eats whole grain bread or cereal, fruits, or vegetables. "Fat" indicates the number of times each week that the respondent eats red meat, cheese, eggs, and butter.

Alcohol use is measured as over two drinks per day. Two or fewer drinks per day may confer some health benefits [14]. The alcohol variable is zero for those respondents with two or fewer drinks and equals the actual number of drinks beyond two.

Exercise minutes per week is calculated as the sum of reported minutes running, brisk walking, swimming, aerobic dance, and other aerobic activities.

Costs are calculated on the basis of the respondent's hospital and doctor visits as well as days spent confined to the home. We use $750 and $65 to value one day in the hospital and one doctor visit. Each day confined to the home is valued at $4 per hour for sixteen hours. The $4 figure is calculated using 40 percent of an annual $20,000 salary (1987 dollars) for the typical retiree prior to retirement. This 40 percent value on leisure time is frequently used in economic studies [15]. The $20,000 figure is only a few dollars more than the mean salary for bank employees nationwide [16].

In the analysis below, costs will be used as a separate explanatory variable in an attempt to control for overall health status. The higher the person's medical costs, the worse his or her health is assumed to be.

Table 2 presents the univariate correlation coefficients and p values for two-tailed tests in parentheses. Reading down each column, a number of interesting results emerge.

Positive correlation coefficients for education are found with exercise, seat belt use, alcohol use, and fiber, and negative coefficients are found with cigarette use, costs, and fat in the diet. However, years of education is statistically significant ($p < .05$) in its positive association with only two habits: exercise and fiber.

Statistically significant ($p < .05$) univariate associations for age include male (positive), cigarettes (negative), fiber (positive), and fat (positive). Statistically significant correlation coefficients with being male include education (positive), age (positive), exercise (positive), seat belts (negative), alcohol (positive), and fiber (negative).

P-values below .05 on univariate coefficients for exercise include education (positive), male (positive), cigarettes (negative), costs (negative), fiber (positive), and fat (negative). The statistically significant ($p < .05$) correlations with cigarettes include age (negative), exercise (negative), seat belts (negative), alcohol

Table 1. Definitions, Means, and Standard Deviations of Variables

Variables	Mean	Standard Deviation
Age	68.527	6.787
Male = 1	.449	.497
Years of *education*	12.936	1.946
Times each week eats *fiber* (Fiber = whole grain bread or cereal, fruits, vegetables)	20.47	8.435
Times each week eats *fat* (Fat = red meat, cheese, eggs, butter, cream, whole milk, low fat milk)	9.07	6.367
Minutes of *exercise* in a typical week	134.06	159.356
Packs of *cigarettes* per day	.118	.358
Percent of times wears *seat belts*	86.569	28.252
Drinks of *alcohol* each day *over 2* (Drink = 1 mixed drink or 1 beer or 1 glass of wine)	.331	1.359
Costs = [(750 × hospital days) + (65 × doctor visits) + (56 × days confined to home during past 6 months)]	$1642.80	$2723.10

(positive), costs (positive), fiber (negative), and fat (positive). Significant univariate correlates of seat belt use include male (negative), cigarettes (negative), alcohol (negative), costs (negative), fiber (positive), and fat (negative). Statistically significant univariate alcohol correlates are male (positive), cigarettes (positive), seat belts (negative), fiber (negative) and fat (positive).

Table 3 presents multiple regression results in which each of the six habits is treated as a dependent variable. Two regressions are reported for each habit: one without and the other with costs entered into the regression. Costs are included to account for current health status. In results available from the authors, an analog measure of overall health status was used in lieu of total costs; results were closely similar.

Two numbers appear in each cell. The first represents the estimated slope and the second the *t*-statistic. The estimated slope is an estimated partial derivative [17]. *T*-statistics over 1.96 are statistically significant in a two-tailed test at the .05 level. *T*-statistics are inversely associated with *p*-values.

For exercise, results for both columns are similar. Age is statistically significant. One more year of age is associated with roughly 1.8 minutes less exercise per week. Being a male is statistically significant; men exercise roughly 29.7 minutes more per week than women. Years of education are not statistically

Table 2. Correlations Between Study Variables
Univariate Correlation Coefficients and (p-values in a two-tailed test)

	Education	Age	Male	Exercise	Cigarettes	Seat belts	Alcohol	Costs	Fiber	Fat
Education										
Age	-.016 (.405)									
Male	.217* (.0001)	.2464* (.0001)								
Exercise	.074* (.0009)	-.038 (.081)	.080* (.0022)							
Cigarettes	-.0285 (.1972)	-.063* (.003)	-.032 (.138)	-.112* (.0001)						
Seat belts	.0064 (.775)	.005 (.806)	-.116* (.0001)	.0418 (.056)	-.076* (.0005)					
Alcohol	.029 (.195)	.018 (.410)	.199* (.0001)	-.017 (.491)	.105* (.0001)	-.102* (.0001)				
Costs	-.037 (.093)	.050 (.021)	.022 (.311)	-.074* (.0007)	.106* (.0001)	-.092* (.0001)	.027 (.221)			
Fiber	.046* (.038)	.063* (.004)	-.108* (.0001)	.122* (.0001)	-.151* (.0001)	.138* (.0001)	-.094* (.0001)	-.045* (.0414)		
Fat	-.0057 (.796)	.046* (.035)	.011 (.597)	-.073* (.0007)	.0757* (.0005)	-.121* (.0001)	.054* (.0145)	.007 (.7439)	-.052* (.018)	

*Indicates statistically significant at the .05 level and two-tailed test.

Table 3. Multiple Regression Analysis of Study Variables

Independent Variables	Dependent Variables, Estimated Coefficients, and (absolute t-statistics)					
	Exercise		Cigarettes		Seat Belts	
	1	2	3	4	5	6
Intercept	148.211*	150.35*	.473*	.458*	74.035*	74.358*
	(3.094)	(3.140)	(4.622)	(4.493)	(8.839)	(8.896)
Age	−1.765*	−1.697*	−.0027*	−.0029*	.127	.146
	(3.161)	(3.034)	(2.241)	(2.467)	(1.278)	(1.465)
Male = 1	29.673*	29.693*	−.0441*	−.0498*	−6.556*	6.510*
	(3.700)	(3.700)	(2.560)	(2.558)	(4.601)	(4.580)
Years of education	3.380	3.314	−.0018	−1.0015	.251	.231
	(1.729)	(1.696)	(.437)	(.372)	(.720)	(.666)
Times each week eats fiber	2.267*	2.255*	−.0051*	.0050*	.338*	.334*
	(5.166)	(5.141)	(5.386)	(5.325)	(4.320)	(4.278)

Times each week eats fat	−.857 (1.476)	−.885 (1.525)	.0026* (2.066)	.0027 (2.162)	.525* (5.115)	−.531* (4.278)
Minutes of exercise each week			−.002* (3.327)	−.002* (3.135)	.0057 (1.387)	−.005 (1.242)
Packs of cigarettes per day	−35.914* (3.327)	−33.971* (3.135)			−3.181 (1.652)	−2.607 (1.351)
Percent of time wears seat belt	.181 (1.387)	.162 (1.242)	−.0005 (1.652)	−.0004 (1.351)		
Drinker of alcohol each day over 2	−1.594 (.597)	1.524 (.571)	.0259* (4.550)	.0254* (4.476)	−1.241* (2.615)	−1.214* (2.565)
Costs		−.002 (1.894)		.00001* (3.941)		−.0008* (3.179)
R^2	.034	.041	.0513	.0591	.0542	.0593
n	1864	1864	1864	1864	1864	1864

*Indicates statistical significance at the .05 level in a two-tailed test.

Independent Variables	Alcohol		Fiber		Fat		Means
	7	8	9	10	11	12	13
Intercept	.933* (2.239)	.927* (2.222)	6.865* (2.728)	6.891* (2.737)	7.371* (3.864)	7.583* (3.968)	
Age	-.006 (1.264)	-.006 (1.296)	.123* (4.220)	.124* (4.235)	.056* (2.529)	.061* (2.713)	68.527
Male	.565* (8.225)	.565* (8.220)	2.599* (6.213)	-2.598* (6.210)	-.336 (1.056)	-.397 (1.235)	.449
Education	-.009 (.547)	-.009 (.538)	.307* (2.995)	.306* (2.987)	.024 (.314)	.0304 (.389)	12.936
Fiber	-.0075* (1.962)	-.0075 (1.955)			.024 (1.364)	-.025 (1.374)	20.47
Fat	.009 (1.826)	.0093 (1.840)	-.042 (1.364)	.042 (1.374)			9.07

28

	(1)	(2)	(3)	(4)	(5)	(6)
Exercise	−.0001	−.0001	.006*	.006*	.0015	−.001
	(.597)	(.571)	(5,166)	(5.141)	(1.652)	(1.525)
Cigarettes	.426*	.421*	−3.038*	−3.017*	.967*	.938*
	(4.550)	(4.476)	(5.386)	(5.325)	(2.255)	(2.162)
Seat belts	−.003*	−.0029*	.0294*	.0292*	−.027*	−.027*
	(2.615)	(2.565)	(4.320)	(4.278)	(5.285)	(5.185)
Alcohol			−.275*	−2.74	.2015	.196
			(1.962)	(1.955)	(1.891)	(1.840)
Costs		.662E-5		−.00003		.00006
		(.571)		(.395)		(1.157)
R^2	.0647	.0649	.0805	.0806	.027	.0287
Sample size	1864	1864	1864	1864	1864	1864
	134.08	.118	85.569	.331	1642.8	

*Indicates statistical significance at the .05 level in a two-tailed test.

significant at the .05 level in a two-tailed test. If a one-tailed test is deemed appropriate, education is statistically significant, however, since the critical $t =$ 1.645 for a p-value of .05 in a one-tailed test.

Fiber is strongly and positively associated with exercise; the t-statistic on fiber is the biggest of all the t-statistics in the exercise regressions. For the exercise results, consumption of one more unit of fiber per week is associated with 2.3 minutes more of exercise per week. A strong and statistically significant correlation is apparent for cigarettes; one more pack per day is associated with thirty-three to thirty-six fewer minutes per week of exercise.

The cigarette smoking results are shown in the next two columns. Age enters negatively and is statistically significant. Older cohorts smoke less. Ten more years of age is associated with smoking 3/100 less of one pack of cigarettes per day. While statistical significance is apparent, clinical or biological significance is weak. Being male is negatively and statistically significant in its association with cigarette use. The men smoked 4/100 less of one pack per day than women, other things being equal. Years of education are not statistically significant in its association with cigarette use in this senior sample. Additional statistically significant correlates in the cigarette columns include fiber (negative), fat (positive), exercise (negative), alcohol drinks over two per day (positive), and costs (positive). Fiber intake is the correlation with the biggest t-statistic in the cigarette columns.

The seat belt results are shown in the next columns. Statistically significant ($p < .05$) multivariate correlates include being male (negative), fiber (positive), fat (negative), alcohol (negative), and costs (negative). Men use their seat belts 6 or 7 percent less often than women. Excessive drinkers are less likely to fasten their seat belts. Four-drinks-a-day drinkers use their belts roughly 5 percent less often than abstainers and light drinkers. The statistically significant results on alcohol suggest that being male and using cigarettes are positively associated with excessive drinking, and that fiber in the diet and seat belt use are negatively associated with excessive drinking. Persons who smoke two packs a day drink roughly one more glass of beer, wine, or liquor per day than persons who don't smoke.

Fiber results appear in columns 9 and 10. Statistically significant ($p < .05$) multivariate correlates of fiber in the diet include age (positive), being male (negative), years of schooling (positive), exercise (positive), cigarette use (negative), seat belts (positive), and alcohol consumption over two per day (negative). Three more years of schooling is associated with one more unit of fiber per week.

Statistically significant ($p < .05$) multivariate correlates of fat in the diet include cigarette use (positive) and seat belt use (negative). One more pack of cigarettes per day is associated with one more time per week eating fat.

Table 4 summarizes many of the results in Tables 2 and 3. The first row of variables indicates one of the six habits. The second and following rows list the first to last "most important" statistically significant correlates of that particular

Table 4. Summary of Statistically Significant Correlation Coefficients (1) and Multiple Regression Coefficients (2)
(Correlates are listed in order of strength of association)

Exercise		Cigarettes		Seat Belts		Alcohol		Fiber		Fat	
1	2	1	2	1	2	1	2	1	2	1	2
Fiber	Fiber	Fiber	Fiber	Fiber	Fat	Male	Male	Cigarettes	Male	Seat belts	Seat belts
Male	Male	Exercise	Alcohol	Fat	Male	Cigarettes	Cigarettes	Seat belts	Cigarettes	Cigarettes	Age
Cigarettes	Cigarettes	Costs	Costs	Alcohol	Fiber	Seat belts	Seat belts	Fiber	Exercise	Exercise	Cigarettes
Education	Education	Alcohol	Exercise	Costs	Costs	Fiber	Fiber	Exercise	Seat belts	Age	
Fat		Male	Male		Alcohol	Fat		Male	Age	Alcohol	
		Age	Age					Alcohol	Education		
		Fat	Fat					Age	Alcohol		
								Education			

habit. "Most important" is determined by the size of the correlation coefficient for univariate associations and the size of the *t*-statistic for multivariate associations. Each habit has two columns of correlates beneath it. The first are drawn from Table 2 (correlation coefficients) and the second from Table 3 (multiple regression results). Consider the first column under exercise. The largest statistically significant univariate correlation coefficient associated with exercise is fiber. The second largest statistically significant univariate correlation from Table 2 is male. In the second column under exercise, the variable explaining exercise with the largest *t*-statistic in Table 3 is fiber. The second largest *t*-statistic is male = 1.

In results available from the authors, an additional "overall health" variable, measured on an analog scale, was added to the regressions and "costs" were deleted. Strikingly similar results were obtained. The inclusion or exclusion of "costs" or the additional "overall health" measure did not affect the statistical significance of other independent variables.

DISCUSSION

This study explores the interrelationships among health habits, education, age, and gender in a large sample of retirees. Because we cannot claim that the sample is representative of all U.S. retirees, this study is descriptive. The great advantages of the sample are the large size and the wealth of information gathered on habits. Our discussion below addresses the four purposes of the study mentioned in the introduction.

Education is widely believed to be a very important predictor of who is and is not likely to practice healthy habits [18-22]. The results above do not support this conclusion in an older retiree sample. Years of schooling achieves statistical significance at the .05 level in a two-tailed test only once: in the fiber regressions in Table 3. Several explanations can be offered for this result.

Bank of America retirees are not a random sample of all U.S. retirees. Bank of America retirees have high socioeconomic status. Years of schooling has a very small standard deviation in these data. Less than 5 percent of the sample had fewer than twelve years of schooling. For the adult American population at large, this figure is roughly 26 percent [23]. The lack of statistical significance of education in these results could be the result of our truncated sample, particularly since the direction of the effect noted is consistent with prior studies. When variation on a variable is truncated it becomes more difficult to achieve statistical significance [24]. Alternatively, this could be a real finding. Callahan and Pincus find a much stronger relation between education and poor health among those with low levels of schooling than those with higher levels of schooling [25]. Our results could, therefore, reinforce those of Pincus and Callahan, since our insignificant education results occur in a sample of relatively well-educated adults. A final explanation could involve the age of the sample. We are not familiar with any similar analyses of habits data with a sample of exclusively retirees. It could be that the influence schooling has is early in life and that by the time the person retires he or she had adopted (or not) healthy habits. Many persons with low education and associated poor health may have already died prior to retirement so that persons with low education who make it to retirement are more likely to have adopted healthy habits sometime during their lives.

The second purpose of this study pertains to whether healthy habits are adopted as a group or if they are traded off, or if they are independent of each other. The evidence strongly supports that found in Breslow and Enstrom [4], Mechanic and Cleary [5], and Wiley and Camache [6]: healthy habits are positively associated with other healthy habits and negatively associated with unhealthy habits. The "trade-off" or "compensating risk" and "null" independence hypotheses are thus rejected.

The third purpose is to look for inter-habit correlations. A number of these correlations merit attention. First, cigarette use and excessive drinking are strongly and positively related. Second, seat belt use and excessive drinking are strongly and inversely related. It is likely that all three behaviors (cigarettes, seat belt use and excessive drinking) are the result of some underlying personality trait such as the ability to delay gratification or tastes for risks [25, 26].

Fiber in the diet appears to be more strongly positively correlated with other healthy habits and inversely correlated with negative habits than any other. The "fiber" variable is clearly deficient when comparing heavy eaters with light eaters since heavy eaters are likely to be fat and consume more of all foods than light eaters. Excess weight is a risk factor for many diseases. One possible solution to this problem would involve controlling for body mass in the analysis. But body mass is not a habit; it is the result of diet, exercise, and genetics. Inclusion of body mass in the analyses would discount the importance of diet and exercise in their associations with other habits and with education, age, and gender. Since this study is designed to investigate habits, body mass is deliberately omitted from the analyses. In lieu of body mass, a measure of fat consumption was included.

Fiber appears at or near the top of "important correlates," more than any other variable in Table 4. Moreover, the R^2s for the fiber regressions are 30 to 200 percent larger than R^2s for the other habit regressions. Habits *as a group* are more strongly correlated with fiber in the diet than with any other single variable. This strong showing for fiber may be the result of the assimilation of preventive medicine information by the public. The public has likely understood the negative consequences of smoking, non-use of seat belts, excessive drinking, inadequate exercise, and fat in the diet for many years. "Fiber" as a health watchword probably only surfaced within the mid-1980s in the minds of the lay public. The persons who now watch fiber in their diet are quick adopters of new preventive medicine practices. They are much more likely than the slower adopters to practice all of the healthy habits and eschew all of the unhealthy habits in Table 3.

As further evidence for this explanation, consider the statistically significant correlation between fiber and education and the statistically significant *t*-statistic on education in the fiber regressions. Wozniak has argued and presented evidence that people with high levels of education are more likely to quickly adopt new technologies than people with low levels of education [27]. The same phenomenon may occur here. The importance of fiber in the diet was a relatively new idea for lay people in the mid-1980s. The more educated may have been more likely to change their habits in response to this new information than the less educated.

Our fourth purpose involves age and gender comparisons. We find that retiree women in this sample are more likely than men to smoke, use seat belts, and eat foods high in fiber. Men are more likely than women to exercise and drink excessively. Apart from the smoking finding, the others are consistent with male/female differences in the literature [28]. The result suggesting that men smoke less than women in these data is curious. It may nevertheless result from selection bias. Male smokers may be more likely to die young than female smokers.

Apart from the curious smoking difference, the results on the other habits conform to those found elsewhere. The negative age and exercise correlation is easily understood: increasing age is a strong predictor of increasing disability which, in turn, is associated with decreased exercise. The statistically insignificant age-seat belt association is at variance with findings from samples with wide age ranges in which age is positively associated with seat belt use. Again, these insignificant results may be due to our sample: the nonusers may be predominately among youth. The inverse and strongly significant finding for cigarette use and age could be the result of selection bias: heavy smokers are less likely to live to enjoy a long retirement than nonsmokers.

Two methodological points bear mentioning. First, R^2s in each regression are relatively low. However, if low R^2s are themselves statistically significant, as ours are in Table 3, we may still legitimately consider each variable's correlation with the dependent variable in all of the multiple regressions reported in Table 3 [29]. Second, because each multiple regression is constructed in the same way with the same explanatory variables, then t-statistics across equations are identical. The t-statistics on fat in the fiber equation are identical to the t-statistics on fiber in the fat regression. This must be true for every paired comparison [30].

Care must be exercised in attempting to generalize these results to other populations. Although the response rate was high, and, although the retirees appear to fairly represent Bank of America retirees, self-selection bias may affect some of the results. Since individual-specific information on people who did not return the questionnaires was not available, econometric self-selection correction techniques could not be permitted [31]. But given that the literature on habits and education is thin (to nonexistent) using large samples of retirees, these results should at least suggest hypotheses to future researchers who might obtain random samples of retirees with detailed information on healthy habits.

The most important findings are:

1. Healthy habits are positively associated with other healthy habits and negatively associated with unhealthy habits. These seniors, on average, do not appear to trade off one healthy habit for an unhealthy one. It, therefore, seems plausible that an underlying desire for health is the principle cause for persons adopting healthy habits.

2. Years of formal schooling do not appear to be strongly correlated with healthy habits in this sample. The weak associations between habits and education level may be due to the limited range of education in the sample: very few of the retirees had less than a high school education. It may also be due to the age of persons in the sample. It could be that education is associated with healthy habits for only the young and middle-aged, and that the poorly educated from older cohorts who live to enjoy retirement may have adopted healthy habits for most of their lives.

3. Fiber consumption is the habit most strongly correlated with all of the others. This result is consistent with the idea that there is a group of health conscious people in the sample who quickly adopt the latest preventive medicine advice [32]. During the late 1980's information on smoking, drinking, seat belt use, and exercise was widespread. Information on the importance of fiber in the diet was, by comparison, relatively new to the public. Persons who attempted to increase their fiber consumption in the 1980s were probably more likely than others to have already stopped smoking, curtailed excessive drinking, frequently used seat belts, and exercised.

Correlates and predictors of healthy habits are receiving increasing attention in the literature. We need additional information on which policies and programs foster health habits both at the individual and societal levels. Bad habits might be like dominoes. We need to know where to intervene. Future research should address, for example, whether people who stop smoking eventually begin to eat more nutritious foods, drink in moderation or not at all, exercise more frequently, and wear seat belts.

REFERENCES

1. N. B. Belloc, Relationship to Health Practices and Mortality, *Preventive Medicine, 2*, pp. 122-147, 1982.
2. N. B. Belloc and L. Breslow, Relationship of Physical Health Status and Health Practices, *Preventive Medicine, 1,* pp. 409-421, 1972.
3. L. S. Robertson, Estimate of Motor Vehicle Seat Belt Effectiveness and Use: Implications for Occupant Crash Protection, *American Journal of Public Health, 66*, pp. 859-864, 1976.
4. L. Breslow and J. E. Enstrom, Persistence of Health Habits and Their Relationship to Mortality, *Preventive Medicine, 9,* pp. 469-483, 1980.
5. D. Mechanic and P. D. Cleary, Factors Associated with the Maintenance of Positive Health Behavior, *Preventive Medicine, 9,* pp. 805-814, 1980.

6. J. A. Wiley and T. C. Camache, Life-style and Future Health: Evidence from the Alameda County Study, *Preventive Medicine, 9,* pp.1-21, 1980.

7. J. K. Langlie, Interrelationships Among Preventive Health Behaviors: A Test of Competing Hypotheses, *Public Health Reports, 94*:3, pp. 216-225, May-June 1979.

8. C. Whipple, Redistributing Risk, *Regulation, 9,* pp. 37-44, 1985.

9. G. J. S. Wilde, The Theory of Risk Homeostasis: Implications for Safety and Health, *Risk Analysis, 2,* pp. 209-225, 1982.

10. R. M. G. Norman, Interrelationships Amongst Health Behaviors, *Canadian Journal of Public Health, 76,* pp. 407-410, November/December 1985.

11. J. P. Leigh, Schooling and Seat Belt Use, *Southern Economic Journal, 37*:3, pp. 321-331, 1990.

12. G. M. Goldbaum, P. L. Remington, K E. Powell, G. C. Hogelin, and E. M. Gentry, Failure to Use Seat Belts in the U.S., *Journal of American Medical Association, 295*:18, pp. 2459-2462, May 1986.

13. SAS Institute, *SAS User's Guide,* Version 5, SAS Institute, Inc., Cary, North Carolina, 1985.

14. A. Klatsky, G. Friedman, A. Siegelaub, and M. Gerard, Alcohol Consumption and Blood Pressure, *New England Journal of Medicine, 296,* pp. 1194-1200, September 26, 1977.

15. E. I. Hatziandreu, J. P. Koplan, M. C. Weinstein, et al. A Cost-Effectiveness Analysis of Exercise as a Health Promotion Activity, *American Journal of Public Health, 78*:11, pp. 1417-1421, November 1988.

16. Bureau of Labor Statistics, *Handbook of Labor Statistics,* Table 42, p.168, Department of Labor Bulletin 2340. U.S. Government Printing Office, Washington, D.C., August 1989.

17. J. P. Leigh, Assessing the Importance of an Independent Variable in Multiple Regression: Is Stepwise Unwise?, *Journal of Clinical Epidemiology, 41*:7, pp. 669-677, 1988.

18. J. P. Leigh, Direct and Indirect Effects of Education on Health, *Social Science and Medicine, 17*:4, pp. 227-234, April 1983.

19. M. Grossman and T. Joyce, Socioeconomic Status and Health: A Personal Research Perspective, in *Pathways to Health: The Role of Social Factors,* J. P. Bunker, D. S. Bomby, and B. H. Kehrer (eds.), The Henry J. Kaiser Family Foundation, Menlo Park, California, 1989.

20. P. Farrell and V. R. Fuchs, Smoking and Health: The Cigarette Connection, in *The Health Economy,* V. R. Fuchs (ed.), Harvard University Press, Cambridge, Massachusetts, pp. 243-254, 1986.

21. W. Rakowski, Personal Health Practices, Health Status, and Expected Control Over Future Health, *Journal of Community Health, 11*:3, pp. 189-203, Fall 1986.

22. D. S. Kenkel, Health Knowledge, Behavior, and Schooling, *Journal of Political Economy,* in press.

23. B. E. Kaufman, *The Economics of Labor Markets and Labor Relations* (2nd Edition), The Dryden Press, San Francisco, California, 1989.

24. G. C. Cain, The Challenge of Segmented Labor Market Theories to Orthodox Theory: A Survey, *Journal of Economic Literature, 14*:4, pp. 1215-1257, December 1976.

25. L. F. Callahan and T. Pincus, Formal Education as a Marker of Clinical Status in Rheumatoid Arthritis, *Arthritis and Rheumatism, 31,* pp. 1346-1357, 1983.

26. J. P. Leigh, Accounting for Tastes: Correlates of Risks and Time Preferences, *Journal of Post-Keynesian Economics, 9*:1, pp. 17-31, Fall 1986.
27. G. D. Wozniak, Human Capital, Information and the Early Adoption of New Technology, *Journal of Human Resources, 22*:1, pp. 101-112, Winter 1987.
28. I. Waldron, What Do We Know About Causes of Sex Differentials in Mortality? A Review of the Literature, *Population Bulletin of the United Nations,* Publication No. 18-1985, 1986.
29. G. S. Maddala, *Introduction to Econometrics*, Macmillan, New York, 1988.
30. A. Goldberger, Reverse Regression and Salary Discrimination, *Journal of Human Resources, 19*, pp. 293-318, Summer 1984.
31. J. J. Heckman and V. J. Hotz, Choosing Among Alternative Nonexperimental Methods for Estimating the Impact of Social Programs: The Case of Manpower Training, *Journal of American Statistical Association, 84:*408, pp. 662-874, December 1989.
32. V. K Smith and W. H. Desvousges, Subjective Versus Technical Risk Estimates: Do Risk Communication Policies Increase Consistency? *Economic Letters, 31*:3, pp. 287-291, 1989.

Chapter 3

SELF-EFFICACY AND DEPRESSIVE SYMPTOMATOLOGY IN OLDER ADULTS: AN EXPLORATORY STUDY

Jennifer Davis-Berman

Self-efficacy theory, as a fairly recent development in social learning literature, suggests the importance of self-efficacy as a cognitive mediator of subsequent behavioral performance. According to Bandura, a self-efficacy expectation reflects an individual's subjective perception of the conviction that he or she can successfully perform or execute a particular behavior [1]. These cognitive expectations have been shown to be common across related or similar situations, creating generalized expectancies [1]. These generalized efficacy expectations can be likened to a pervasive frame of reference within which competency is assessed, regardless of objective reinforcement.

In an attempt to examine the validity of self-efficacy as a behavioral predictor, the majority of previous research has focused on anxiety disorders. These studies have indicated that self-efficacy is a consistent predictor of behavioral performance [2, 3]. Recent researchers have investigated self-efficacy as a mediating variable in the following areas: smoking cessation [4-6], achievement in children [7-10], career development [11-12], and athletic performance [13-15].

Very little work has examined the application of the self-efficacy theory to the older adult population, or to the investigation of either clinical depression or depressive symptomatology in this population. Initial attempts in these areas have either failed to focus on the self-efficacy construct [16], or have not included any measure of depression or depressive symptomatology [17]. Recent studies have considered self-efficacy as a mediator in both social support and depression [18, 19]. However, these studies failed to objectify self-efficacy or the assessment of depression.

DEPRESSION

Traditionally, studies of depression focus on two basic data sources: diagnosed clinical depression and self-reports of depressive symptomatology [20]. It has been argued that data from these different sources describe two distinctly different types of depression [21]; on the other hand, it has also been argued that these differences relate simply to the severity of symptoms, rather than to underlying etiology [22]. Due to the more extensive data-gathering required for the diagnosis of clinical depression, community-based investigations tend to favor the examination of depressive symptoms [20].

Although depressive symptomatology may not be more prevalent among older adults than among other age groups [23], its impact on the mental health status of older adults is significant. Studies suggest that between 11 percent and 54 percent of community-residing older adults suffer from noticeable depressive symptomatology [24, 25], and that the prevalence is even higher among institutionalized populations [26].

SELF-EFFICACY

Based on previous research, it can be suggested that self-efficacy expectations play an important role in mediating a variety of behaviors and mood states [1-17]. Importantly, they have also been shown to predict social support and subsequent depressive symptomatology in older adults [19].

Given our society's generally negative attitudes toward elderly adults, one could suggest that the self-efficacy construct may be especially applicable to the elderly. It can be argued that negative perceptions of self-efficacy may be related to depressive symptomatology in older adults, and that due to the rather marginal status of this population group, their vulnerability to this relationship may be heightened. This relationship between cognitions and subsequent mood and behavior is not unlike the learned helplessness formulation of depression, except that self-efficacy expectations are independent of outcome expectancy and causal attribution [27].

The purpose of the present study was to explore the relationship between self-efficacy and depressive symptomatology among community-residing older adults. Consistent with previously developed scales, the self-efficacy construct was divided into three components: general, social, and physical self-efficacy. This division not only serves to objectify the self-defficacy construct, but the examination of physical self-efficacy may be expecially relevant to older adults, due to the numerous physical changes and losses associated with the aging process.

The present exploratory study was based on the following predictions:

1. Levels of self-efficacy (as measured by general, social, and physical self-efficacy scales) would be related to depressive symptomatology.
2. Based on the numerous physical losses and changes associated with age, and the relationship between physical illness and depressive symptomatology [28], a strong relationship between physical self-efficacy and depressive symptoms was expected.
3. Self-efficacy expectations (as measured by general, social, and physical self-efficacy scales) would be significant predictors of depressive symptomatology.

METHOD

Respondents

Two hundred respondents were randomly selected from a sampling frame of 1,241 members of the Golden Age Senior Citizen's Center in Xenia, Ohio. This center serves the older adult population in Greene County, Ohio. A total of 200 respondents were successfully interviewed by telephone. Of those contacted, twenty-four refused to participate in the study, yielding an 89 percent response rate. However, those who refused to participate were replaced with respondents in the sample who agreed to the interview.

Seventy-nine percent of the respondents were female, 52 percent of whom were unmarried at the time of the study. Ages of the respondents ranged from sixty to ninety-two, with a mean age of seventy. The modal income category for the sample was $0-$10,000, with 88 percent of the respondents reporting that they were not employed at the time of the interviews.

Data Collection

Data were collected by the primary investigator and one trained research assistant. All potential respondents were contacted by telephone. Those who agreed to participate were read data-collection instruments in an interview which lasted approximately twenty-five minutes.

Instrumentation

Depressive symptomatology was assessed using Form E of the Depression Adjective Checklist. This instrument contains thirty-four single-word adjectives. These adjectives were read to the respondents who were asked to indicate the adjectives that described their moods at the time of the interview [29, 30]. Examples of these adjectives include: unhappy, lonely, peaceful, hopeless, and lucky [30]. The DACL was scored in the direction of health to correspond with the self-efficacy scales; high scores represent fewer depressive symptoms. The possible range of scores on the inventory was zero (high number of depressive symptoms) to thirty-four (low number of depressive symptoms).

The depression adjective checklist has been shown to have high internal consistency reliability (.91 for depressive adjectives, and .82 for nondepressive adjectives), and alternate form reliability (.82). The DACL has also been shown to be highly correlated with other measures (Beck Depression Inventory, $r = .56$; depression scale of the MMPI, $r = .49$). Finally, both the concurrent validity and the discriminant validity of the DACL have been shown to be high [31-35] .

Self-Efficacy

Perceptions of self-efficacy were assessed through the use of an existing self-efficacy inventory [36], and a physical self-efficacy inventory [37]. The self-efficacy inventory consists of two scales: general and social self-efficacy. Originally, these scales were designed with likert-type response categories. However, in the present study, it was decided that these categories were too cumbersome for use with the telephone survey method, and therefore response categories were collapsed into dichotomous yes/no categories. Examples of some of the items from the general and social self-efficacy scales include: I am a self-reliant person; I feel insecure about my ability to do things; it is difficult for me to make new friends; and I do not handle myself well in social gatherings [37]. Possible scores on the general self-efficacy scale ranged from 0-17; the scores on the social self-efficacy scale ranged from 0-6, with low scores suggesting low levels of perceived self-efficacy.

Although relatively recent in their development, these scales have been shown to have high reliability (Alpha = .86, general self-efficacy; Alpha = .71, social self-efficacy), construct validity, and criterion validity [36] .

The physical self-efficacy inventory consists of twenty-two items. The possible score range was 0-22, with low scores suggesting low levels of perceived self-efficacy. Examples of some of the items from this scale include: I have excellent reflexes, I have poor muscle tone, and I take pride in my ability in sports [37].

Test-retest and internal consistency reliabilities have been found to be high with this scale (.80 and .82 respectively). In addition, both construct and criterion validity were found to be high [37].

Finally, the following demographic information was collected: marital status, income category, employment status, gender, and age.

RESULTS

The scores on the DACL ranged from 9 to 34, with a mean of 30.8 and a standard deviation of 4.4. In accordance with the traditional scoring of the DACL, this reported mean was transformed into a sample mean of 4.09, suggesting low levels of endorsement of depressive symptoms.

Scores on the general self-efficacy scale ranged from 0 to 17, with a mean of 14.5, and a standard deviation of 3.4, suggesting fairly high levels of general self-efficacy. Scores on the social self-efficacy scale ranged from 0 to 6, with a mean of 4.17, and a standard deviation of 1.9, again suggesting fairly high levels of social self-efficacy. Finally, scores on the physical self-efficacy scale ranged from 0 to 22, with a mean of 15.4, and a standard deviation of 4.4, with high scores suggesting high physical self-efficacy.

Following this descriptive analysis, Pearson correlations were performed to examine potential relationships between general, social, and physical self-efficacy and scores on the DACL. The following relationships were found to be statistically significant: general self-efficacy and DACL ($r = .54$), social self-efficacy and DACL ($r = .29$), and physical self-efficacy and DACL ($r = .55$).

In an attempt to determine the strength of self-efficacy expectations as predictors of DACL scores, a stepwise multiple regression procedure was run. The results indicated that physical self-efficacy was the most significant predictor of DACL score, accounting for 30 percent of the variance in DACL scores ($F = 85.58$, $R^2 = .301$). As may be seen in Table 1, general self-efficacy was identified as the second strongest predictor, accounting for an additional 9.37 percent of the variance ($F = 64.45$, $R^2 = .395$).

Table 1. Standardized Regression Coefficients
and Zero-Order Correlations[a]

Independent Variables	Depression Adjective Checklist	
	Beta	r
Physical Self-Efficacy	.39*	.55*
General Self-Efficacy	.36*	.54*
Social Self-Efficacy	.02	.29*
R^2	.40	

[a] Zero-order correlations are reported in the positive direction due to the aforementioned scoring transformations performed on the DACL.
   * $p < .01$.

DISCUSSION

Difficulties in the interpretation of the present results arise from the lack of refinement of the measurement instruments used. The DACL does not provide guidelines within which to interpret the scores; for example, scores indicating low, medium, and high amounts of depressive symptomatology are not provided. The present mean of 4.0 on the DACL, however, can be compared to a mean of 7.54 using Form E in the National Depression Survey [31]. Clearly, respondents in the present study endorsed significantly fewer depressive adjectives than did those in the general population.

Given this rather large disparity, the representativeness of the sample, and the validity of the telephone survey method must be questioned. Although the study sample was drawn from a relatively large sampling frame, it can be argued that this sample was biased. Those older adults who join senior citizen's centers, regardless of actual participation in the centers, may be less prone to either experiencing or acknowledging negative mood states than the general population of older adults.

Finally, although the telephone survey method may be quite appropriate for use with older adults, its ability to control for social desirability bias has been questioned [38]. It is quite possible that respondents were reluctant to acknowledge the negative adjectives in this context.

In much the same way, no guidelines for interpretation of the self-efficacy scales have been established, with the exception of high scores suggesting high levels of self-efficacy. The present results suggest that respondents reported fairly high levels of self-efficacy. As predicted, however, physical self-efficacy was seen to have the lowest mean of the self-efficacy scales.

As predicted, general, social, and physical self-efficacy were significantly correlated with DACL scores, suggesting that strong perceptions of self-efficacy were related to the absence of depressive symptomatology. This relationship, as expected, was most strong between physical self-efficacy and the DACL.

Support for the self-efficacy construct as a predictor of reported depressive symptomatology was gained through the multiple regression analysis. In this analysis, physical self-efficacy was identified as a significant predictor of depressive symptoms, accounting for 30 percent of the variance in DACL scores.

The significance of physical self-efficacy as a predictor of self-reported depressive symptoms may be especially relevant to older adults, as this population group has been shown to be more vulnerable to chronic illness [39]. Additionally, it has been well established that the stress of physical illness may encourage the development of depressive symptoms [28]. In addition to these direct linkages between illness and depressive symptoms, the present results suggest the importance of a cognitive mediator, physical self-efficacy.

It can be suggested that the subjective assessment of physical well-being and general physical competence is a powerful variable independent of the objective physical status of the individual. This finding suggests important avenues for both future research and practice.

The role of physical self-efficacy as a cognitive variable should be further explored by looking at the relationship between physical self-efficacy, perceived physical health status, and actual physical health status. In an attempt to further define these relationships, respondents could be asked not only to rate their perceived physical self-efficacy, but may also be asked to perform a behavior which relates to that specific physical dimension. In this way, the relationship between physical self-efficacy and actual behavior may be more accurately assessed.

Explorations of these relationships could also serve to enrich practice with older adults. Based on these exploratory findings, perceived physical self-efficacy appears to be an important construct which may be used therapeutically in a few important ways. Group or individual work with middle-aged and older adults may focus on restructuring our interpretations of the normal physical changes associated with aging. This could be done in an attempt to strengthen physical self-image to compensate for areas of actual physical loss. Finally, it would be interesting to determine if group work geared toward increasing physical functioning, dexterity, and flexibility could actually influence physical self-efficacy and depressive symptomatology. If this were true, we would not only increase our physical competence for its own sake, but possibly improve our mental status as well.

REFERENCES

1. A. Bandura, Toward a Unifying Theory of Behavioral Change, *Psychological Review, 84,* pp. 191-215, 1977.
2. A. Bandura, N Adams, and J. Beyer, Cognitive Processes Mediating Behavioral Change, *Journal of Personality and Social Psychology, 35,* pp. 125-139, 1977.
3. A. Bandura, N. Adams, A. Hardy, and G. Howells, Tests of the Generality of Self-Efficacy Theory, *Cognitive Therapy and Research, 4,* pp. 39-66, 1980.
4. M. Condiotte and E. Lichtenstein, Self-Efficacy and Relapse in Smoking Cessation Programs, *Journal of Consulting and Clinical Psychology, 49,* pp. 648-658, 1981.
5. C. DiClemente, Cognitive Processes in Intimate Conflict: Efficacy and Learned Helplessness, *The American Journal of Family Therapy, 9,* pp. 35-44, 1981.
6. J. Prochaska, Self Change Processes, Self-Efficacy and Self Concept in Relapse and Maintenance of Cessation of Smoking, *Psychological Reports, 51,* pp. 983-990, 1982.
7. D. Schunk, Modeling and Attributional Effects on Children's Achievement: A Self-Efficacy Analysis, *Journal of Educational Psychology, 73,* pp. 93-105, 1981.
8. D. Schunk, Effects of Effort Attributional Feedback on Children's Perceived Self-Efficacy and Achievement, *Journal of Educational Psychology, 74,* pp. 548-556, 1982.
9. V. Wheeler and G. Ladd, Assessment of Children's Self-Efficacy for Social Interactions with Peers, *Developmental Psychology, 18,* pp. 795-805, 1982.

10. B. Zimmerman and J. Ringle, Effects of Model Persistence and Statements of Confidence on Children's Self-Efficacy and Problem Solving, *Journal of Educational Psychology, 73*, pp. 485-493, 1981.
11. G. Hackett and N. Betz, A Self-Efficacy Approach to the Career Development of Women, *Journal of Vocational Behavior, 18*, pp. 326-339, 1981.
12. K. Taylor and N. Betz, Applications of Self-Efficacy Theory to the Understanding and Treatment of Career Indecision, *Journal of Vocational Behavior, 22*, pp. 63-81, 1983.
13. C. Lee, Self-Efficacy as a Predictor of Performance in Competitive Gymnastics, *Journal of Sport Psychology, 4*, pp. 405-409, 1982.
14. A. Meyers, R. Schleser, and T. Okwumabua, A Cognitive Behavioral Intervention for Improving Basketball Performance, *Research Quarterly for Exercise and Sport, 53*, pp. 344 -347, 1982.
15. R. Weinberg, D. Yukelson, and A. Jackson, Effect of Public and Private Efficacy Expectations on Competence Performance, *Journal of Sport Psychology, 2*, pp. 340-349, 1980.
16. C. Pearson and M. Gatz, Health and Mental Health in Older Adults: First Steps in the Study of a Pedestrian Complaint, *Rehabilitation Psychology, 27*, pp. 37-50, 1982.
17. P. Hogan, The Effect of Physical Activity on the Self-Efficacy, Leisure Satisfaction, and Subjective Well Being of Older Adults, *Dissertation Abstracts International, 42*, p. 3449, 1982.
18. C. K. Holahan, C. J. Holahan, and S. S. Belk, Adjustment to Aging. The Roles of Life Stress, Hassles, and Self-Efficacy, *Health Psychology, 3*, pp. 5-328, 1984.
19. C. K. Holahan and C. J. Holahan, Self-Efficacy, Social Support, and Depression in Aging: A Longitudinal Analysis, *Journal of Gerontology, 42*, pp. 65-68, 1987.
20. S. Nolen-Hoeksema, Sex Differences in Unipolar Depression: Evidence and Theory, *Psychological Bulletin, 2*, pp. 259-282, 1987.
21. R. A. Depue and S. M. Monroe, Learned Helplessness in the Perspective of the Depressive Disorders: Conceptual and Definitional Issues, *Journal of Abnormal Psychology, 87*, pp. 3-20, 1978.
22. R. M. A. Hirschfeld and C. K. Cross, Epidemiology of Affective Disorders: Psychosocial Risk Factors, *Archives of General Psychiatry, 39*, pp. 35-46, 1982.
23. L. Srole and A. K. Fischer, The Midtown Manhattan Longitudinal Study vs. "The Mental Paradise Lost" Doctrine, *Archives of General Psychiatry, 37*, pp. 209-221, 1980.
24. E. H. Hare and G. K. Shaw, Mental Health on a New Housing Estate, *Maudsley Monograph 12*, Oxford University Press, Oxford, 1965.
25. D. C. Leighton, *The Character of Danger*, Basic Books, New York, 1963.
26. D. Blazer, The Epidemiology of Mental Illness in Later Life, in *Handbook of Geriatric Psychiatry*, E. W. Busse and D. G. Blazer (eds), Van Nostrand Reinhold, New York, 1980.
27. L. Y. Abramson, M. E. D. Seligman, and J. D. Teasdale, Learned Helplessness in Humans: Critique and Reformulation, *Journal of Abnormal Psychology, 87*, pp. 49-74, 1978.
28. G. Klerman, Problems in the Definition and Diagnosis of Depression in the Elderly, in *Depression and Aging: Causes, Care, and Consequences*, L. Breslau and M. Haug (eds.), Springer Publishing Company, New York, pp. 3-19, 1983.

29. B. Lubin, *Depression Adjective Checklist,* Educational and Industrial Testing Service, San Diego, 1967.

30. E. Levitt and B. Lubin, *Depression: Concepts, Controversies and Some New Facts,* Springer Publishing, New York, 1975.

31. A. Roth and B. Lubin, Factors Underlying the Depression Adjective Checklists, *Educational and Psychological Measurement,* pp. 383-387, 1981.

32. B. Lubin and P. Himelstein, Reliability of the Depression Adjective Checklists, *Perceptual and Motor Skills, 43,* pp. 1037-1038, 1976.

33. B. Lubin, *Manual for the Depression Adjective Checklists,* Educational and Industrial Testing Service, San Diego, 1967.

34. B. Lubin, *Manual for the Depression Adjective Checklists,* Educational and Industrial Testing Service, San Diego, 1981.

35. F. C. Byerly, *Comparison between Inpatients, Outpatients, and Normals on Three Self-Report Depression Inventories,* unpublished doctoral dissertation, Western Michigan University, 1979.

36. M. Sherer, J. Maddux, B. Mercandante, S. Prentice-Dunn, B. Jacobs, and R. Rogers, The Self-Efficacy Scale: Construction and Validation, *Psychological Reports, 51,* pp. 663-671, 1982.

37. R. Ryckman, H. Robbins, B. Thornton, and P. Cantrell, Development and Validation of a Physical Self-Efficacy Scale, *Journal of Personality and Social Psychology, 42,* pp. 891-900, 1982.

38. D. Dillman, *Mail and Telephone Surveys: The Total Design Method,* Wiley and Sons, New York, 1978.

39. E. Pfeiffer and E. Busse, Mental Disorders in Later Life. Affective Disorders: Paranoid, Neurotic, and Situational Reactions, in *Mental Illness in Later Life,* E. Busse and E. Pfeiffer (eds.), Garamond/Pridemark, Baltimore, 1973.

Chapter 4

DEPRESSION, DEMENTIA, AND SOCIAL SUPPORTS

Sally R. Esser
and
Peter P. Vitaliano

As the aged population increases [1], the diagnosis of dementia and its differentiation from other causes of global cognitive impairment becomes more challenging. The diagnosis of dementia is important both in terms of the etiology of the disease and the cost of long-term care [2]. Although a complete medical "work-up" for dementia may include expensive tests such as EEG and CT scan, the cost of these tests is much less than the cost of long-term institutionalization [3]. The diagnosis of irreversible dementia may result in decreased medical attention to the patient and increased mortality [4]. The diagnosis of dementia is particularly difficult because other factors contribute to the clinical presentation; these include normal aging, the effects of other diseases, and social factors.

It is important that the primary care physician recognize the interrelations of dementia, depression, and social supports in order to provide a more complete evaluation of the elderly patient with non-organic cognitive impairment. This chapter will clarify the usage of the terms dementia, depression, pseudodementia, and social support before examining each of these and their relation to elderly individuals with cognitive impairment.

Dementia is diagnosed by inclusion and exclusion criteria, namely 1) loss of intellectual abilities to such extent that social and occupational functioning is compromised, 2) memory impairment, 3) unclouded state of consciousness, 4) one of the following: impaired abstract thinking or judgment, disturbances of higher cortical functioning (aphasia, apraxia, agnosia, constructional difficulty) or personality change and 5) evidence from history, physical examination, or lab of a specific organic factor deemed responsible for the disturbance or exclusion of causes other than organic mental disorders [5]. This definition of dementia is clinical and does not differentiate between reversible and irreversible causes. Dementia is a syndrome with many potential causes and contributing factors. Other organic mental disorders which must be considered in the differential diagnosis include normal aging changes, delirium (in which there is clouding of consciousness), schizophrenia, and depression.

The diagnostic criteria for depression include dysphoric mood and at least four of the following: weight/appetite change, insomnia/hypersomnia, psychomotor changes, loss of pleasure in usual activities, fatigue, feelings of worthlessness/guilt, diminished ability to think/concentrate, and thoughts of death. There must be no evidence of schizophrenia, paranoid disorders, delusions, hallucinations, or uncomplicated bereavement processes [5].

Pseudodementia is a term that has been used to describe functional psychiatric disorders that present a clinical picture of dementia [6]. Depressive pseudodementia indicates that a depressive illness is producing dementia-like symptoms [4].

Social support has been defined as an "enduring pattern of continuous or intermittent ties that play a significant part in maintaining the psychological and physical integrity of an individual over time. . . ." [7]. It is characterized by 1) psychological and emotional help and guidance, 2) task sharing, and 3) the provision of extra materials and skills. It may be regarded as information which leads the individual to believe that he or she is loved, valued, and part of a network of communication and mutual obligation [8] .

DEMENTIA

Five percent of the American population over age sixty-five has severe dementia and is unable to care for itself; an additional 10 percent has mild or moderate dementia. Fifty to 80 percent of elderly nursing home residents have the diagnosis of dementia [2, 9]. Once dementia is diagnosed, survival time is approximately three years, as opposed to nine years for non-demented age matched controls [3]. Alzheimer's disease is estimated to account for 50-75 percent of all dementias, and multi-infarct dementia for 15-20 percent [9, 10] . Other irreversible causes are much less common. Treatable causes such as depression, drug toxicity and hypothyroidism, account for approximately 20 percent of all dementias [11, 12]. Although patients with "reversible" dementia improve with treatment, Larson et al. found these patients generally do not achieve normal intellectual functioning and will often present an irreversible dementia at a later period of time [12].

Patients with reversible dementia have been found to have a shorter duration of symptoms, less cognitive impairment (as determined by the Mini-Mental State Examination), more prescribed medications, and fewer abnormal elements in their mental status examinations [12]. The natural history of irreversible dementia is characterized by deterioration, although the time course is highly variable [1, 13]. In a patient presenting a possible dementia, it is important to obtain a thorough history from the patient and the family, and to perform a physical examination, including neurological and psychological testing. The neurological examination traditionally includes maneuvers to elicit primitive reflexes, such as the glabellar, snout, and grasp reflexes. However, in a recent study comparing age-matched Alzheimer's patients and normal participants, no correlation was found between psychometric testing and the presence of primitive reflexes [14]. Detection of asterixis (flapping tremor) can be helpful because it is a sign of metabolic disease and is not found in Alzheimer's disease, multi-infarct dementia, or depression [11]. Psychometric tests useful in evaluating dementia include the Mini-Mental State Examination (MMS) [15, 16] and the Dementia Rating Scale (DRS) [17-20]. The DRS is a relatively new measure that has been used effectively in assessing various types of cognitive impairment (attention, conceptualization, memory, etc.) in dementia patients. Vitaliano et al. have shown that the DRS is a reliable and clinically useful measure not only for discriminating between severity and dementia levels, but also for predicting functional decline over time [19, 20].

In a prospective outpatient study, the only laboratory tests that proved to be of general value in evaluating dementia were the complete blood count, the SMA-12, and thyroid function tests [12]. Although the CT scan and EEG may rule out a focal problem, they do not specifically diagnose Alzheimer's disease [10]. CT scan was found to be of value only in a subset of patients, namely those with 1) history of an acute deterioration and 2) either recent onset (less than one year) or mild dementia (MMS score greater than 20). In patients with either 1) no history of acute deterioration or 2) prolonged duration of symptoms (over three years) and severe dementia (MMS score less than 16), CT scan was not found to be helpful. Using these criteria to determine the use of CT scan, no less than 96 percent of all important CT findings would be detected with 95 percent certainty [12]. Such criteria must be used with flexibility and allowing for clinical judgment.

DEPRESSION

The role of depression in dementia has many facets. Some authors suggest that depression may be a symptom of dementia, although it is difficult to determine whether depression appearing early in the course of a dementia is actually a direct effect of the pathology of dementia or is a reaction by the patient to the memory impairment and other cognitive symptoms. Below, we will discuss both depression as a coexisting phenomenon in dementia and the possible clinical presentation of depression as dementia.

Depression is considered the most common mental illness suffered by elderly people. In this respect, 25 percent of all suicides occur in people over the age of sixty-five [21]. Unfortunately, the diagnosis of depression in this age group is complicated by normal changes of aging and changes in behavior and cognition due to physical illnesses [22]. Elderly people are more likely to complain of physical symptoms than emotional or mood changes. The impaired concentration, memory loss, and functional deficits which are characteristic of depression in all age groups are often accentuated in elderly patients. In addition, elderly people are at greater risk for severe depression, in which their refusal to eat, drink, move about, or even communicate can become life-threatening [21].

Normal changes in aging that do not necessarily indicate depression include decreased energy level and motor/sensory function, and social withdrawal as a result of physical disabilities or transportation difficulties [22]. Aging can also result in losses of family, friends, jobs, status, and home. Depression in older adults is often said to be a result of these losses, particularly the loss of family and friends. Traditionally, such social supports as family and friends have been viewed as "buffers" against the effects of stress, including changes in finances, health, and social status. Aneshensel and Stone have found that both stress and lack of social supports have direct effects on depression, and that social support in itself provides a positive effect on mental health [23]. Depression alone can cause distress or weaken social supports [23, 24].

Murrell et al. found that in a population of over fifty-five years of age, depression increased with age, poverty, and poor health, while it decreased with education and size of one's dwelling place. Divorced, separated or widowed respondents were more likely to experience depression than married or single participants. Of the variables studied, physical health had the strongest association with depression [25]. In contrast, Steur et al. found no association between physicians' ratings of health and depression as measured by the Zung Self-Rating Depression Scale (SDS), but did find a significant association between fatigue and depression. Steur et al. were not able to find reliable data that an elderly population would respond to the SDS similarly to a group of younger adults, and their study reflects problems with the use of this measure with elderly groups [26].

The etiology of the depressive episode is important to determine. Drug-induced depressions are common in elderly patients [21]. Depression may be secondary to a physical illness which can be treated [21, 22]. Moreover, depression may occur as a concurrent but separate entity with other diseases, and as such, it needs to be treated separately. Diagnosis of depression is generally made by a careful history, physical, and mental-status exam, with particular attention to the criteria described previously.

Differentiating depression from dementia is a task often necessary in both clinical and research work. In fact, the history and symptoms are usually different in these two entities. Depression is marked by a rapid onset, stable and apathetic mood, poor self image, and self reproach, and is generally self-limited and reversible with medication, electroconvulsive therapy, or psychotherapy. Dementia, as described earlier, has an insidious onset, labile mood, normal self image, and is chronic and progressive [1]. Depressed elderly patients have been found to perform slightly below or better than average on assessments of memory, implying little overall cognitive impairment, while primarily demented patients have exhibited some cognitive impairment. The MMS has been found to differentiate between demented patients, depressed patients with cognitive dysfunction, and depressed patients without cognitive dysfunction. In particular, the MMS has demonstrated that only depressed patients over sixty years of age present with cognitive impairment. Patients with more severe depression also tended to have greater cognitive impairment [15, 16]. Thus, it is important to evaluate both the mood level and cognition involved, as they may be interrelated or represent separate problems.

DEPRESSION AND DEMENTIA

Depression has been estimated to be as high as 20 percent in patients with chronic illness. Riefler et al. examined the etiology of cognitive impairment in elderly outpatients. Of their eighty-eight patients, 3 percent had cognitive impairment due to depression only, 20 percent had impairment due to depression and dementia, and 77 percent were impaired as a result of dementia. Patients with more severe cognitive deficits were significantly less likely to be depressed. Age did not affect the incidence of depression, and men and women were found to have similar rates of depression. The question has been raised whether a greater incidence of depression in less demented patients implies a protective effect of depression against the characteristic deterioration of dementia, but such long-term follow-up has not yet been performed [27].

Memory impairment and other cognitive changes have been observed in both depressed elderly patients and demented elderly patients. In patients with coexistent dementia and depression, one would expect worsened cognitive function. Patients with dementia and depression exhibited significantly lower Full Scale I.Q. scores than patients with dementia alone, but differences in short-term memory were not found to be significant. Scores on the Wechsler Adult Intelligence Scale and the Wechsler Memory Scale have not been significantly different in demented depressed and demented nondepressed patients [28].

PSEUDODEMENTIA

The final relationship between depression and dementia that this chapter will discuss is the role depression may play in the clinical presentation of dementia. The literature on pseudodementia addresses two primary issues. First, is the concept of pseudodementia valuable in describing and diagnosing patients, or does it simply blur the interaction between dementia and psychiatric illnesses, particularly depression? Second, how does one differentiate pseudodementia from an irreversible dementia?

The term pseudodementia is usually credited to Kiloh, who presented ten case studies in which the "diagnosis of dementia was entertained, but had to be abandoned" [6]. Although Kiloh's case studies did not involve elderly people and not all of his participants returned to a pre-morbid level of functioning, the term pseudodementia continues to be used both as a description and a diagnosis. The appeal of the term pseudodementia arises from the assumptions that 1) a patient may be incorrectly diagnosed as demented and thus be denied appropriate therapeutic measures, and 2) a patient has to be either depressed or demented.

Wells has supported the use of the term pseudodementia, citing clinical differences between pseudodementia and dementia, involvement of psychiatric disorders other than depression, and the lack of a significant association between symptoms and brain damage. Wells based his observations on ten cases involving patients under the age of seventy who often had other underlying brain disorders [29]. Wells developed clinical criteria which could be used to differentiate pseudodementia and dementia. Patients with pseudodementia generally are aware of their cognitive deficits, can provide a history of their illness, and are upset by their cognitive impairment. They are more likely to answer questions with "I don't know" than provide a "near miss" response. A "near miss" response is typical of an organic deficit. Patients with pseudodementia may have memory loss during specific periods, unimpaired concentration and attention, and less deterioration at night [1, 29].

Shraberg presented a case study in which a depressive episode was superimposed on an early dementia; he suggested that "the concept of dementia and depression occurring as parallel and interrelated processes in the senium" is more helpful than the concept of pseudodementia [30]. Others have recognized that reversible dementia-like symptoms thought to be pseudodementia may represent a subclinical dementia that has been made more pronounced by a depressive episode [31].

Folstein and McHugh have found that in depressed patients over the age of sixty-five, scores on the MMS were often within the range of scores typical of patients with known dementia; however, these scores returned to normal levels with treatment of the depression. In addition, these patients usually had a rapid onset of symptoms typical of depression and frequently had a history of affective disorders. Folstein and McHugh suggested that the term "dementia syndrome of depression" be used rather than "pseudodementia" [16].

Reifler has argued that pseudodementia is not a useful term, for three primary reasons: pseudodementia ignores the possibility of coexistent dementia and depression, suggesting "mutually exclusive pathological processes;" the term does not allow for coexistent reversible and irreversible processes; and contrary to its original function as a descriptor, "pseudodementia" has been interpreted as a diagnostic category [32].

Additional problems with the term "pseudodementia" are that 1) a widely accepted diagnostic criteria for pseudodementia has not been formulated, partly because of diverse clinical presentations in reported case studies, 2) there is little data on the frequency of pseudodementia, and 3) there have been no studies on neurobiological dysfunction in pseudodementia [33].

SOCIAL SUPPORT

A relationship between social support and illness has long been recognized. Poor social support is positively associated with increased risk for both physical and psychiatric illness in the general population, and this association increases for people over the age of fifty [34]. The presence of an intimate confidant has been shown to reduce both the incidence and severity of depressive illness after a major life event [7]. Elderly people lacking a confiding relationship have been found to be at higher risk for depressive illnesses than elderly people with such a relationship [35].

Gallo has described the dimensions of social support networks in terms of size, frequency, density, distance, content, intensity, homogeneity, duration, and directedness. Of these dimensions, he found size, homogeneity, density, and distance to be positively related to health status. Frequency of contact and duration of the relationship did not significantly correlate with health [36]. Connor et al. found that neither the number nor frequency of interactions were important for elderly individuals. Quality, rather than quantity, of interactions determined the degree of satisfaction or positive effect attained [37].

It is not clear whether a poor support system causes a person to adapt to stressors poorly, thereby increasing physical and psychiatric illness, or whether physical and/or psychiatric illness prevent a person from forming an adequate support system [8, 38-40]. Social support may directly affect mental well-being and/or act as a buffer during times of stress. Williams et al. have found that the negative effects of life events and physical illness did not vary with the level of social support, implying that life events and social supports may not interact directly. Instead, social supports seem to have positive value for an individual, regardless of the severity level of the individual's life events [41]. Not all life events are undesirable, and their level of desirability or undesirability differs according to each individual. Events considered undesirable are more highly correlated with psychological status than events in general. Desirable events have only a low correlation with psychological status [42]. Of the most common life events of elderly individuals, major medical events and retirement are followed by more significant changes and decreased life satisfaction than are retirement of a spouse, widowhood, or departure of a child. Widowhood appeared to increase social interaction for most of the elderly individuals studied [43, 44].

Feelings of helplessness have been related to depression and may contribute to withdrawal, physical disease, and even death. Such factors as improvement in affect, activity, and mental alertness have been observed in elderly patients with responsibilities and decision-making roles, whereas increased debilitation has been observed with the loss of responsibility and the need to make decisions [45]. Long-term follow-up at eighteen months revealed better general health and lower mortality rates in the group with responsibility as opposed to the "helpless" groups

[46]. Institutionalized elderly people are particularly at risk for learned helplessness, thus increasing their level of disability and depression [45, 47]. Providing responsibility and inclusion in a supportive network is clearly only a partial answer to a complex problem.

DISCUSSION

Relationships among dementia, depression, and aging are only beginning to be understood. Defining "normal" aging is a difficult task, given the high percentage of elderly people who must also deal with social isolation, one or more physical illnesses, losses of many types, and other stressors. Changes in intellectual functioning secondary to normal aging need to be defined before one can evaluate the effects of disease or psychosocial factors. Many of the psychometric tests used to measure cognitive function may be inappropriate for elderly patients. Although many of the tests have been developed for school children or college students, a significant number of elderly patients may not have a similar educational background. Moreover, these tests often do not measure the ability of the respondent to function in the "real world" [48]. As Steur et al. have found, elderly members of a patient population may respond differently to a test than other members of that population [26].

The literature of pseudodementia is plagued both by problems in defining the condition and the relatively small group of patients who serve as a description of such a condition. The original descriptive use of the term may be useful in differentiating psychiatric etiologies of reversible dementia-like syndromes from medical causes such as thyroid disease and pernicious anemia. However, at present, there are multiple problems with the use of the term pseudodementia: 1) it is used as a diagnosis rather than a description, 2) it lacks both accepted diagnostic criteria and prevalence data, 3) it lacks research on the pathophysiology of the condition, and 4) it blurs interrelations between depression and dementia. As the literature on coexisting depression and dementia illustrates, the interrelation between depression and dementia clearly extends beyond cause-and-effect relationships. The role of depression in exacerbating a mild, previously subclinical dementia is just beginning to be studied.

In general, the social support and stress literature has not separated the direct effect of stressors on social support from the interactive buffering effect of social supports on health in the presence of stressors [40]. Nor has the effect of social supports alone on physical and mental health been adequately studied [40, 41].

The social support literature has not clearly explained the role of social resources in response to stressors, in part because of theoretical and methodological problems. Researchers have defined social support in many ways, without achieving a standard operational term, developing valid and reliable indicators of social support, or considering its multidimensionality [40]. The amount, type, and source of support, as well as the structure of the support network, must be considered [36, 37, 40]. Thoits has suggested that the definition of social supports reflects both socioemotional aid (affection, sympathy, understanding, esteem) and instrumental aid (advice, information, help with family or work responsibilities, financial aid). This allows researchers to examine structural properties such as size, density, accessibility, kinship-reliance, frequency of contact, stability, and functional properties such as perceived amount and adequacy of support [40]. With clarification of the terminology and methodology, research such as that described by Gallo [36] and Connor et al. [37] can be extended to better explore the complex interactions of stressors, illness and social supports.

As was described above, specific aspects of social support seem especially important to elderly individuals. Unfortunately, much of the literature focuses on hospitalized or institutionalized patients. Indeed, although they represent the vast majority of aged people in this country, relatively few studies have dealt with elderly outpatients.

The problem of interpreting causality arises in much of the literature reviewed here and will probably not be easily resolved. Does social isolation lead to cognitive impairment, or has there been a long-standing psychological problem leading to a poorly maintained social support system? Does dementia depress the elderly person, who senses cognitive dysfunction, or are these independent but coexisting entities? The term "pseudodepression" has been offered as a description for dementias that appear as depression [49].

CONCLUSIONS

Although geriatric workers are now beginning to understand the empirical relationships discussed in this chapter, the issues that arise clinically involve the diagnostic differentiation between dementia and depression and the treatment of elderly patients with cognitive deficits of non-organic etiology. In the early 1960s, Kiloh summarized the relationship of dementia to psychiatric illness by recognizing that 1) depression must be considered in the differential diagnosis of dementia-like symptoms, 2) symptoms of brief duration or a relapsing course were not characteristic of dementia, 3) a normal EEG is suggestive of a diagnosis other than dementia, and 4) psychometric testing may not be adequate for differentiating groups [6]. We now recognize that both mood and cognition must be evaluated to determine the extent of dysfunction, and that an evaluation of the patient's social network may provide clues to both etiology and prognosis of the impairment. Together with the history of onset and progression of symptoms, the MMS may lead to methods for differentiating between depression and dementia. Familiarity with using the MMS or DRS and their regular use with elderly patients may be of value to primary care physicians. The criteria for the use of CT scan are valuable, particularly in the evaluation of patients with MMS scores between sixteen and twenty and/or unclear histories of onset and duration. Finally, the possibility of coexisting dementia and depression and the role of depression in causing dementia-like symptoms must be considered in elderly patients with cognitive impairment.

Further research needs to be done to clarify the relationships and interactions which have been discussed. More objective criteria for both depression and dementia, in addition to clinical history and presentation, need to be formulated. Psychological and cognitive tests need to be specifically developed for elderly patients. Studies need to utilize elderly outpatients, the so-called healthy elderly, as well as those in institutions and hospitals. Participants should include individuals over seventy-five since this population is increasing and may differ from individuals age sixty to seventy-five. Criteria to separate dementia into mild, moderate, and severe categories should be tested for validity and implications for prognosis and treatment. Further research on the coexistence of dementia and depression, including the role of depression in early dementia and the potential for the return of cognitive function, is vital to our understanding of dementia and depression. As noted above, research on the 1) prevalence of, 2) criteria for, and 3) pathophysiology of pseudementia must be done to elucidate the role of psychological illness in dementia syndromes. Finally, research must be continued on the relationship between social supports and health, specifically the contributions of families and institutions to the mental health of the elderly population.

REFERENCES

1. S. Gershon and S. Herman, The Differential Diagnosis of Dementia, *Journal of the American Geriatric Society, 305,* S58, 1982.
2. R. N. Butler, Charting the Conquest of Senility, *Bulletin of the New York Academy of Medicine, 58,* p. 362, 1982.
3. K. Steel and R. Feldman, Diagnosing Dementia and its Treatable Causes, *Geriatrics, 3,* p. 79, 1979.
4. B. Kramer, Depressive Pseudodementia, *Comprehensive Psychiatry, 23,* p. 538, 1982.
5. *American Psychiatric Association: Diagnostic and Statistical Manual of Mental Disorders* (3rd Edition), Washington, D.C., 1980.
6. L. G. Kiloh, Pseudodementia, *Acta Psychiatrica Scandinavica, 37,* p. 336, 1961.
7. J. Gelein, The Aged American Female: Relationships Between Social Support and Health, *Journal of Gerontological Nursing, 6,* p. 69, 1980.
8. R. J. Turner, Social Support as a Contingency in Psychological Well-being, *Journal of Health and Social Behavior, 22,* p. 357, 1981.
9 K. Kosik, and J. Growden, Aging, Memory Loss and Dementia, *Psychosomatics, 23,* p. 745, 1982.
10. W. G. Rosen, Update on Dementia, *Journal of the American Medical Womens Association, 37,* p. 214, 1982.

11. Task Force Sponsored by National Institute of Aging: Senility Reconsidered, *Journal of the American Medical Association, 244,* p. 259, 1980.
12. E. B. Larson, B. V. Reifler, H. J . Featherstone et al., Dementia in Elderly Outpatients: A Prospective Study, Clinical Research, 31, p. 642A, 1983.
13. L. Heston, A. Mastri, V. E. Anderson et al., Dementia of the Alzheimer's Type, *Archives of General Psychiatry, 38,* p. 1085, 1981.
14. W. Koller, S. Glatt, R. Wilson et al., Primitive Reflexes and Cognitive Function in the Elderly, *Annals of Neurology, 12,* p. 302, 1982.
15. S. Cavanaugh and R. M. Wettstein, The Relationship Between Severity of Depression, Cognitive Dysfunction and Age in Medical Inpatients, *American Journal of Psychiatry, 140,* p. 495, 1983.
16. M. F Folstein and P. R. McHugh, Dementia Syndrome of Depression, in *Alzheimer's Disease: Senile Dementia and Related Disorders* (Aging, Vol. 7), R. Katzman, R. D. Terry, and K. L. Bicks (eds.), Raven Press, New York, p. 87, 1978.
17. M. Coblentz, S. Mattis, L. H. Zingesser et al., Presenile Dementia: Clinical Evaluation of Cerebrospinal Fluid Dynamics, *Archives of Neurology, 29,* p. 299, 1973.
18. S. Mattis, Mental Status Examination for Organic Mental Syndrome in the Elderly Patient, in *Geriatric Psychiatry,* R. Bellack and B. Karasu (eds.), Grune and Stratton, New York, 1976.
19. P. Vitaliano, A. Breen, M. Albert et al., Memory, Attention and Functional Status in Community Residing Alzheimer Type Dementia Patients and Optimally Healthy Aged, *Journal of Gerontology, 39,* p. 58, 1984.
20. P. Vitaliano, A. Breen, J. Russo et al., The Clinical Utility of the Dementia Rating Scale for Assessing Alzheimer Patients, *Journal of Chronic Disease, 37,* p. 743, 1984.
21. M. Blumenthal, Depressive Illness in Old Age: Getting Behind the Mask, *Geriatrics, 4,* p. 34, 1980.
22. C. Gaitz, Identifying and Treating Depression in an Older Patient, *Geriatrics, 38,* p. 42, 1983.
23. C. Aneshensel and J. Stone, Stress and Depression: A Test of the Buffering Model of Social Support, *Archives of General Psychiatry, 39,* p. 1392, 1982.
24. J. Flaherty, F. M. Gaviria, E. Black et al., The Role of Social Support in the Functioning of Patients with Unipolar Depression, *American Journal of Psychiatry, 140,* p. 473, 1983.
25. S. A. Murrell, S. Himmelfarb, and K. Wright, Prevalence of Depression and its Correlates in Older Adults, *American Journal of Epidemiology, 117,* p. 173, 1983.
26. J. Steur, L. Bank, E. J. Olsen et al., Depression, Physical Health and Somatic Complaints in the Elderly: A Study of the Zung Self-Rating Depression Scale, *Journal of Gerontology, 35,* p. 683, 1980.
27. B. Reifler, E. Larson, and R. Hanley, Coexistence of Cognitive Impairment and Depression in Geriatric Outpatients, *American Journal of Psychiatry, 139,* p. 623, 1982.
28. A. R. Breen, E. Larson, B. V. Reifler et al., Cognitive Performance and Functional Competence in Coexisting Dementia and Depression, *Journal of the American Geriatric Society, 32,* p. 132, 1984.
29. C. E. Wells, Pseudodementia, *American Journal of Psychiatry, 136,* p. 895, 1979.

30. D. Shraberg, The Myth of Pseudodementia: Depression and the Aging Brain, *American Journal of Psychiatry, 135,* p. 601, 1978.
31. J. M Himmelhoch, R. Auchenback, and C. A. Fuchs, The Dilemma of Depression in the Elderly, *Journal of Clinical Psychiatry, 43,* p. 26, 1982.
32. B. V. Reifler, Arguments for Abandoning the Term Pseudodementia, *Journal of the American Geriatric Society, 30,* p. 665, 1982.
33. E. D. Caine, Pseudodementia, *Archives of General Psychiatry, 38,* p. 1359, 1981.
34. G. Andrews, C. Tennant, D. Hewson et al., The Relation of Social Factors to Physical and Psychiatric Illness, *American Journal of Epidemiology, 108,* p. 27, 1978.
35. E. Murphy, Social Origins of Depression in Old Age, *British Journal of Psychiatry, 141,* p. 135, 1982.
36. F. Gallo, The Effects of Social Support Networks on the Health of the Elderly, *Social Work in Health Care, 8,* p. 65, 1982.
37. K. A. Connor, E. A. Powers, and G. L. Bultena, Social Interaction and Life Satisfaction: An Empirical Assessment of Late-Life Patterns, *Journal of Gerontology, 34,* p. 116, 1979.
38. S. Henderson, P. Duncan-Jones, H. McAuley et al., The Patient's Primary Group, *British Journal of Psychiatry, 132,* p. 74, 1978.
39. S. Henderson, A Development in Social Psychiatry: The Systematic Study of Social Bonds, *Journal of Nervous and Mental Disease, 168,* p. 63, 1980.
40. P. A. Thoits, Conceptual, Methodological and Theoretical Problems in Studying Social Support as a Buffer Against Life Stress, *Journal of Health and Social Behavior, 23,* p. 145, 1982.
41. A. W. Williams, J. E. Ware, and C. A. Donald, A Model of Mental Health, Life Events and Social Supports Applicable to General Populations, *Journal of Health and Social Behavior, 22,* p. 324, 1981.
42. D. P. Mueller, D. W. Edwards, and R. M. Yarvis, Stressful Life Events and Psychiatric Symptomatology: Change or Undesirability?, *Journal of Health and Social Behavior, 18,* p. 307, 1977.
43. E. Palmore, W. P. Cleveland, J. B. Nowlin et al., Stress and Adaptation in Later Life, *Journal of Gerontology, 34,* p. 841, 1979.
44. J. A. Kohen, Old But Not Alone: Informal Social Supports Among the Elderly by Marital Status and Sex, *Gerontologist, 23,* p. 57, 1983.
45. E. J. Langer and J. Rodin, The Effects of Choice and Enhanced Personal Responsibility for the Aged: A Field Experiment in an Institutional Setting, *Journal of Personality and Social Psychology, 34,* p. 191, 1976.
46. J. Rodin and E. J. Langer, Long Term Effects of a Control Relevant Intervention with the Institutionalized Aged, *Journal of Personality and Social Psychology, 35,* p. 897, 1977.
47. J. Avron and E. Langer, Induced Disability in Nursing Home Patients: A Controlled Trial, *Journal of the American Geriatric Society, 30,* p. 397, 1982.
48. J. Avorn, Biomedical and Social Determinants of Cognitive Impairment in the Elderly, *Journal of the American Geriatric Society, 31,* p. 137, 1983.
49. R. Morstyn, G. Hochanadel, E. Kaplan et al., Depression vs. Pseudodepression in Dementia, *Journal of Clinical Psychiatry, 43,* p. 197, 1982.

Chapter 5

SOCIAL INTERACTION AND DEPRESSION IN ELDERLY INDIVIDUALS

Ken J. Rotenberg
and
Jocelyn Hamel

It has been widely recognized that depression is a serious problem in elderly individuals. Epidemiological research suggests that depression is evident in over 30 percent of elderly individuals in institutions and, when assessed by symptom checklists, between 10 percent and 45 percent of elderly individuals in the community [1]. Conceptually and empirically, depression is negatively related to life satisfaction, morale, and well-being [2]. The present study was designed to investigate the potential social causes, as opposed to biological and genetic causes, of depression in elderly individuals [3].

THE QUANTITY OF SOCIAL INTERACTION

Some of the social causes of depression in elderly individuals are suggested by "Activity Theory" [4]. This theory postulates that elderly persons must replace lost activities and roles if morale and life satisfaction are to be maintained. A number of hypotheses have been derived from Activity Theory [5, 6]. One of these is that the quantity, and hence amount of frequency, of social interaction positively contributes to morale and negatively contributes to depression in elderly persons.[1] In support of this hypothesis, researchers have found that elderly individuals'

---

[1]The Activity Theory does not strictly suggest that only the quantity of social interaction causes depression in the elderly. For example, on the basis of this theory, researchers have proposed and found that life satisfaction in the elderly is associated with the frequency of interactions with friends [6].

self-reports of the amount and frequency of their social contacts, is positively correlated with their contentment, morale, and life satisfaction [7], and negatively correlated with their psychosocial impairment and depression [8, 9]. This hypothesis was investigated in the present study.

THE QUALITY OF SOCIAL INTERACTION

Some authors have argued that the *quality* of social interaction is a more important cause of depression in elderly individuals than is the *quantity* of social interaction (e.g., [10]). The quality of social interaction has been conceptualized by Beckman as the subjective or perceived level of satisfaction with social interaction [10], and by Snow and Crapo as emotional bondedness to a given person(s), referred to as a confidant [11]. The research has provided support for the hypothesized importance of the quality of social interaction for depression in elderly individuals. Beckman found that elderly women's well-being was correlated with their ratings of the *satisfaction* with the amount and quality of their social interaction [10]. Snow and Crapo found that well-being in elderly medical patients was positively correlated with their scores on an Emotional Bondedness Scale that comprised their self-reported relationship to a given person(s) (potential confidants) in terms of the experience of emotional support, mutual sharing of intimacies, and feelings of positive affect [11]. In these studies, well-being was assessed by composite scores that included either one or both of self-rated life satisfaction and depression.

THE METHODOLOGICAL PROBLEM

A fundamental problem with the research on depression in elderly individuals is that it is largely limited to correlational methods because of the ethical difficulties with the alternative—the experiment. For obvious ethical reasons, researchers would not engage in experimental studies that would, or could potentially, increase depression in elderly individuals. As a result, researchers are limited in conclusions about causation and can at best describe their correlational findings in terms of the "potential causes" of depression.

There is an aspect of the problem with the correlational method in the above research, however, that can be overcome without ethical difficulty. Observed correlations can be due to mediators between two variables and it is very likely that that accounts for the observed correlation between depression and the quality of social interaction. There are two distinct reasons for arriving at this conclusion. First, both variables in the research are self-rated; correlations between such measures are often the result of individuals' mediating evaluative sets. Second, there is a likely candidate for a mediating evaluative set, that of the "negative life view," which has been linked to depression and to self-rated quality of social interaction. It has been observed that the more individuals are depressed, the more they adopt a negative life view that is manifested in their evaluations of the quality of their social relationships [12, 13]. Simply, those who are depressed feel negative about life and hence often feel that "no one cares" about what they say or do. The seriousness of this methodological problem depends on the objectives of the research. If researchers wish to conclude that depression is associated with elderly individuals' *own views* of the quality of their social interaction, as was the objective of Beckman's study [10], then the mediational evaluative set is not that much of a problem. However, if researchers wish to conclude that depression is associated with an independently defined quality of social interaction pattern in elderly individuals then the mediational evaluative set is a serious problem. This appeared to be the objective of Snow and Crapo's study [11].

RESOLUTION IN THE PRESENT STUDY

The present study was designed to resolve the mediational problem by determining whether depression in elderly individuals is correlated with the quality of social interaction when it is assessed by a measure that does *not* depend on the elderly individuals' evaluative view of their social relationships. The method employed in the study drew upon the research on self-disclosure in young adults. It has been found that young adults show the reciprocity of self-disclosure; the intimate self-disclosure of one individual is met by a self-disclosure of equal intimacy of another [14, 15]. As evidence for this process, Jourard and his colleagues have used variations of a round-robin method in which the young adults/peers reported the intimacy of their self-disclosures to each other [14, 16, 17]. It was found that in nursing·and university students, there is a correlation between their reported intimacy of self-disclosure to peers (disclosure output) and their peers' reported intimacy of self-disclosure to them (disclosure input).

A question that can be posed is whether elderly individuals, as a group, show reciprocity of self-disclosure. Although this was addressed in the present study, its focus was on individual differences in the reciprocity of self-disclosure. Specifically, reciprocity of highly intimate self-disclosures is an important part of the "confidant" relationships described by Snow and Crapo as the quality of social interaction [11]. The self-disclosure research methods provided a means of assessing the presence of that communication pattern and relationship. As part of a round-robin method, the elderly individuals reported the intimacy of their self-disclosure to each other. This yielded measures of the extent to which:

a. each elderly individual made intimate self-disclosures to their peers;
b. they received intimate self-disclosures from their peers; and
c. therefore, whether they had relationships characterized by reciprocity of high intimate self-disclosures.

The resulting "reciprocally intimate relationship" measure was not dependent on the elderly individuals' *evaluative* view of their social relationships and therefore that mediator was not a plausible cause of a correlation with depression. Guided by the theory and research by Snow and Crapo [11], it was expected that depression would be negatively correlated with the extent to which the elderly persons had reciprocally intimate relationships.

It was necessary in the present study to limit testing to a small group of elderly individuals because the round-robin testing method required that many of the persons were familiar with *each other*. For this reason, researchers who have used round-robin methods have tested relatively small samples of individuals, such as nine [17]. Although the round-robin method is limited in this fashion, it does provide extensive and detailed information about social relationships.

One additional issue dealt with in the present study was the validity of the self-reports of intimate self-disclosures. Jourard and Landsman found evidence for the validity of that measure by a correlation between the individuals' reported disclosure to their peers and the individuals' estimates of how much those peers knew about them [17]. The problem with this procedure is that each individual provided both reports. The correlation may have resulted from the individuals' attempts to maintain consistency. A validity check procedure that avoided this problem was employed in the present study and it was based on the principle of assessing the correlation between reports from different sources. The elderly individuals reported their disclosure to peers, and the peers (others) reported their knowledge of the elderly individuals. This, as well as other validity checks, were employed in the present study.

It should be emphasized that the present study was not designed to determine whether the quality is, or is not, *more* important than quantity as cause of depression in elderly individuals. The position taken was that depression is related to both the quantity and quality of social interaction, although in *different* ways. The present study was designed to investigate the hypothesis that depression is negatively correlated with both the quantity and quality of social interaction. The relationship between the two social interaction domains was investigated as well.

Depression Measure

Depression in elderly individuals was assessed in the present study by the Zung Self-Rating Depression Scale which has been used for that purpose in other research [18]. Investigation of the properties of this scale has led to the identification of separate somatic and psychological symptoms of depression and their corresponding subscales [19]. Using this distinction, researchers have been found that somatic, but not psychological, symptoms of depression increase with age across adulthood [20], and are correlated with physician rated health in elderly individuals [21]. This distinction was of interest in the present study to the extent that it was expected that *psychological* depression is related to the quality and quantity of social interaction. Unfortunately, it was not feasible in the study to consider this distinction, primarily because the somatic and psychological symptoms subscales appear to be correlated with each other, as well as with the Zung total scale score [21]. These relations were problematic, particularly in this study, because the small sample size did not permit statistical separation of the subscales. Also, the somatic symptoms subscale is small (typically two items) and the psychometric properties of it for a small sample as well were uncertain; making correlations with it difficult to interpret. The smallness of the somatic subscale and its correlation with the total score suggested, however, that the total scale score could serve as a reasonable estimate of the psychological symptoms of depression.

METHOD

Subjects

A total of forty-two elderly individuals participated in the study. The twenty-three elderly individuals who received the complete testing were eighteen female and five male residents from the same senior citizen home. The mean age of the males was 84.6 years and of the females was 82.2 years. As part of the round-robin procedure, nineteen other elderly individuals received partial testing. Of those, twelve were residents of the home and seven were not residents.

Measures

On the Demographic Information Checklist, the elderly individuals were posed a series of questions regarding their: age; gender; marital status; length of widowhood (if appropriate); former occupation; length of retirement; education; current yearly income (ranging from 1—less than $5,000 to 5—above $20,000); self-rated health and self-rated eyesight (both ranged from 1—extremely poor to 5—extremely good); and length of residence in the home.

On the Social Interaction Scale the elderly individuals were required to rate how often they see or hear from each of seven categories of persons [10]. The seven categories were:

1. children;
2. neighbors (with other residents identified separately);
3. other friends (with other residents identified separately);
4. other relatives;
5. young people they felt particularly close to;
6. people they associated with in group activities; and
7. any other people (e.g., counselor, doctor).

The Self-Disclosure Index, developed by Miller, Berg, and Archer, was used to assess intimate self-disclosure [22]. The elderly individuals were posed with eleven intimate topics and asked about their disclosure of those to familiar individuals (targets). (The topics are shown in Appendix A.) While this scale has been established and used with young adults, it contained topics that were broad enough to apply to, and be used by, elderly individuals. For example, some of the topics were: "My deepest feelings" and "What is important to me in life." Also, another topic, "Things I have done in the past," was uniquely added to the scale because of its presumed importance for the elderly. The elderly individuals rated each item from one—discussed not at all, to five—discussed fully and completely.

The Knowledge of Others Index was derived from the Self-Disclosure Index. It included the same topics but the elderly individuals completed the scale in terms of what knowledge they had of each target person. They judged each item on a five-point scale ranging from one—know not at all to five—know fully and completely.

The Zung Self-Rating Depression Scale consisted of twenty items designed to assess depressive symptomatology [18]. The elderly individuals were administered nineteen our of the twenty items. The item "I still enjoy sex" was excluded because the directors of the home thought it was too personal; this item has been excluded by other researchers as well [2].

Procedure

Through the matron of the residence, elderly individuals were obtained who spoke English as a first language and who had the ability to see and hear without difficulty. The elderly individuals were tested individually in two one-hour sessions, held approximately one week apart. During the first session the persons were administered the: Demographic Information Checklist, the Social Interaction Scale, and the Self-Disclosure Index. During the second session the persons were administered the: Zung Self-Rating Depression Scale and the Knowledge of Others Index.

In the administration of the Self-Disclosure Index, the individuals were initially asked to identify up to four persons whom they had talked to frequently during the last month. Three of the persons were to be living within the residence, and the fourth person could live either inside or outside of the residence. The option of choosing a person outside the residence was guided by Cohen and Rajkowski's study, in which it was found that elderly individuals frequently have friends outside of their residence [23]. The persons whom the elderly individuals identified as "disclosure targets" were contacted, and asked to participate in the study. This was undertaken without much difficulty because over 60 percent of those who were were identified as disclosure targets were already participants (see the validity check). Also, 85 percent of those identified were contacted and tested. The disclosure targets were tested only on the Self-Disclosure Index and the Knowledge of Others Index. The disclosure targets who were residents were tested face-to-face, while those who were not residents were tested over the phone. Throughout the following description of the study, "elderly individuals" will be used to denote those who received the complete testing, while "disclosure targets" will be used to denote those who received the partial testing. This is descriptive only, since as part of the round-robin method many "elderly individuals" were "disclosure targets."

RESULTS

Demographic Data

A number of demographic characteristics of the elderly individuals were obtained and the means and standard deviations of those are shown in Table 1. They provide a detailed description of the sample.

Coding of the Measures

Quantity of Social Interaction

Following the procedure used by Beckman, a total frequency of social interaction score was calculated by summing the frequencies of interaction across the seven person categories [10]. The frequency score was multiplied to yield an expected interaction over a year period. The focus of the study on peer-resident interaction, prompted the similar calculation of two other frequency scores:

Table 1. Means and Standard Deviations of the
Demographic Characteristics of the Subjects

| Demographic Characteristics | Statistic | |
	Mean	Standard Deviation
Length of stay in residence	5.96 (years)	4.57
Length of marriage	40.83 (years)	18.06
Length of widowhood	10.22 (years)	9.57
Number of children	2.30	2.57
Years of education	8.52	2.45
Income	1.61	0.84
Length of retirement	16.91 (years)	9.34
Length of spouse's retirement	10.78 (years)	10.21
Self-rated health	2.04	0.88
Self-rated eyesight	2.26	1.25

a. the frequency of interactions with peers that comprised the reported interaction with neighbors and other friends; and
b. the frequency of interactions with residents that comprised the interaction with the same person categories but only those who were identified as fellow residents.

The Self-Disclosure Index yielded one measure of the quantity of social interaction, that of the number of people the elderly individuals reported they talked to frequently—the number of disclosure targets. This measure ranged from zero to four.

Quality of Social Interaction

Each elderly individual's ratings were summed across all eleven topics and disclosure targets identified. That amount was divided by the corresponding numbers of topics and disclosure targets to yield an average intimacy of disclosure *output* score. In addition, the different disclosure targets' ratings on all eleven topics of their disclosure to *each* elderly individual were summed. That amount was divided by the number of topics and disclosure targets to yield an average intimacy of disclosure *input* score. The reciprocity of the disclosure was calculated by subtracting the intimacy of disclosure input score from the intimacy of disclosure output score. The smaller the absolute number, the greater the match and the greater the reciprocity. (The reciprocity of disclosure score was reversed in direction for analysis purposes.)

Whether the elderly individual had reciprocally intimate relationships was calculated by the combined use of the intimacy of disclosure output/input and the reciprocity of disclosure measures. The one-third of the elderly individual sample who had the highest intimacy of disclosure output and input, *and* had the highest reciprocity of disclosure, were identified as those having reciprocally intimate relationships and were assigned a two in the analyses. The remaining elderly individuals were considered as not having reciprocally intimate relationships and were assigned a one in the analyses.

Depression

The Zung Self-Rating Depression Scale raw scale scores ranged from nineteen to seventy-six. They were converted to the SDS index in which the higher the score, the greater the severity of depression [18].

Validity Check

A validity check was implemented for the number of disclosure targets. The validity check was based on the assumption that conversations are largely mutual and therefore if individual X reports that s/he talked to target Y frequently, then Y will report that s/he talked to individual X frequently, as well. There was an overall 63 percent agreement between those reports, providing support for the validity of the number of disclosure targets measure.

A validity check was implemented for the intimacy of disclosure output measure. This was assessed by the correlation, across the elderly individuals, between an individual's intimacy of disclosure output to a given disclosure target and that disclosure target's knowledge of the individual. The correlation was low ($r(40) = .15$). A correlation in which the disclosure target's knowledge of the individual was expressed as a proportion of the target's overall knowledge of all individuals was higher ($r(40) = .23$), although it was not statistically significant. The disclosure target's tendency to conclude that s/he knows others appeared to have confounded the initial correlation.

Correlational Analyses

The correlations among the measures are shown in Table 2. The correlational analyses yielded mixed support for the hypotheses. Contrary to expectation, depression was not correlated with the majority of the measures of the quantity of social interaction. The expected correlation was found, however, between depression and the number of disclosure targets ($r(21) = -.43, p < .05$).

The frequency measures of the quantity of social interaction were derived from a common set of data. For this reason, in part, the total frequency of social interaction was correlated with the frequency of social interaction with peers measure ($r(21) = .98, p < .01$) and the frequency of social interaction with residents measure ($r(21) = .95, p < .01$); which, similarly, were correlated with each other ($r(21) = .97, p < .01$).

A negative correlation was expected between depression and the quality of social interaction. Contrary to expectation, there was a positive correlation between depression and the reciprocally intimate relationships measure ($r(21) = .52, p < .05$).

There were some correlations among the quality of social interaction measures that were used to construct the reciprocally intimate relationship measure. The reciprocity of disclosure measure was negatively correlated with both the intimacy of disclosure output and input measures ($r(21) = -.51, p < .05$ and $r(21) = -.53, p < .01$, respectively). These findings were due to the fact that the greater the intimacy of the disclosure output or input, the more likely there was a mismatch between the two, and hence the less likely there was exact reciprocity.

Evidence for reciprocity of self-disclosure rested on obtaining a correlation between the intimacy of disclosure output and the intimacy of disclosure input. The correlation between those measures was not significant and approached zero.

Some correlations were found between the measures of the quantity and quality of social interaction. The disclosure intimacy output measure was positively correlated with the total frequency of social interaction ($r(21) = .48, p < .05$) and the frequency of interaction with peers ($r(21) = .42, p < .05$).

Table 2. Correlations Among the Variable Measures

		The Measures (By Number)							
Variable	Measure	2	3	4	5	6	7	8	9
Depression	1. SDS Index	-.13	-.10	-.02	-.43*	-.12	.12	.26	.52*
Quantity of Social Interaction	2. Total Interaction		.98**	.95**	.24	.48*	.01	-.41	-.13
	3. Peer Interaction			.97**	.28	.42*	-.10	-.34	-.03
	4. Resident Interaction				.21	.39	-.05	-.36	-.03
	5. Number of Disclosure Targets					-.11	-.43*	.11	-.13
Quality of Social Interaction	6. Intimacy of Disclosure Output						.20	-.51*	.11
	7. Intimacy of Disclosure Input							-.53**	-.15
	8. Reciprocity of Disclosure								.32
	9. Reciprocally Intimate Relationships								

Note: All dfs = 21.

* $p < .05$.
** $p < .01$.

DISCUSSION

The findings yielded support for the validity of the number of disclosure targets; there was an agreement between the elderly individuals' and targets' identification of those whom they talked to frequently. The findings did not yield support for the validity of the intimacy of the disclosure output measure. The correlation between the intimacy of the elderly individuals' disclosure to the targets and the targets' knowledge of them, were not statistically significant. As noted, one of the factors affecting the correlation appeared to be the targets' assumed overall knowledge of others. In addition, the failure to find the expected correlation may be due to the fact that persons' knowledge of another individual may not be solely a function of that individual's disclosure to them. Rather, considerable information may be gained through shared friends and through "gossip." In the future, researchers should find a viable means of assessing the validity of the intimacy of disclosure measure.

A number of studies have found that the quantity of social interaction, as assessed by self-reported frequency of social interaction, is positively correlated with measures of well-being and negatively correlated with depression in elderly individuals [9]. The present study failed to yield a correlation between depression and conventionally used quantity of social interaction measures. However, the study *did* yield a significant correlation between depression and the number of disclosure targets measured reflecting the number of individuals the elderly individuals stated they "talked to" frequently. As mentioned, there was support for the validity of this measure. These findings point to the importance of social conversation as a potential cause of depression in elderly individuals. It may be that elderly individuals become depressed, not because they lack frequent social interaction per se, as has often been proposed, but more specifically because they lack frequent social contacts in which they can *converse*.

Previous researchers have found that depression is negatively correlated with the quality of social interaction, in the form of self-reported "confidant" relationships [11]. The present study was designed to determine whether that correlation would be observed when the quality of social interaction was assessed by a measure that did not depend on elderly individuals' evaluative views of their social interaction. Contrary to the hypothesis derived from the previous research, a positive correlation was found between depression and the measure of having reciprocally intimate relationships. This finding is particularly interesting because depression was not correlated with the intimacy of disclosure measures or the reciprocity of disclosure measure, all of which were used to determine the presence of reciprocally intimate relationships. The observed correlation was an unique and independent one.

One plausible interpretation of this finding is that the more the elderly individual is depressed, the more s/he has friends who exchange *negative* communications, such as complaints. The potential causal relationship here is complex. It may be that depression initially causes the elderly individual to form reciprocally intimate relationships because of the need to share feelings. It may be the case, though, that the social relationship serves to maintain depression because of the negativity of the exchange. These hypotheses warrant further investigation. In addition, the difference between these and previous findings lend support to the initial conclusion that a negative life view mediated the previous correlations between depression and self-rated quality of social relationships.

Unlike young adults, elderly individuals as a group did not show evidence for the reciprocity of self-disclosure. A zero order correlation was found between the elderly individuals' intimacy of disclosure output to peers and their intimacy of disclosure input from peers. One account of this finding is yielded by Selman and Selman, who have proposed that the ability to engage in "mutual" perspective taking is necessary for reciprocal intimacy patterns [24]. Elderly individuals have been found to show poor perspective taking skills and it may be this that prevents them from showing the reciprocity of self-disclosure [25].

Some relationships between the measures of the quality of social interaction and the quantity of social interaction were found. Notably, the frequencies of total and peer interactions were correlated with the intimacy of disclosure output. This may be due to the tendency for elderly individuals who frequently interact with peers to disclose considerable amount of intimate information to them.

The present findings provide a rather interesting picture of the correlates of depression in elderly individuals. Depression in elderly individuals was negatively correlated with having peers with whom they talk to frequently, but unexpectedly, positively correlated with having reciprocally intimate relationships. Furthermore, elderly persons did not show the reciprocity of self-disclosure. These findings were obtained, however, on an "old-old" mixed-sex sample of elderly individuals who were living in a nursing home. In the future, researchers should investigate the generalizability of the findings to other elderly samples varying in age, sex composition, and living conditions. This would provide further information on the relation among depression, communication patterns, and social relationships in elderly individuals.

APPENDIX A: The Eleven Intimate Topics

01. My personal habits.
02. Things that I have done which I feel guilty about.
03. Things I wouldn't do in public.
04. My deepest feelings.
05. What I like and dislike about myself.
06. What is important to me in life.
07. What makes me the person I am.
08. My worst fears.
09. Things I have done which I am proud of.
10. My close relationships with other people.
11. Things I have done in the past.

REFERENCES

1. D. Blazer, *Depression and Aging: Causes, Care, and Consequences*, L. D. Breslau and M. R. Haug (eds.), Springer, New York, pp. 30-50, 1983.
2. J. N. Morris, R. S. Wolf, and L. V. Klerman, Common Themes among Morale and Depression Scales, *Journal of Gerontology, 30*:2, pp. 209-215, 1975.
3. J. M. Davis, N. L. Segal, and G. K. Spring, *Depression and Aging: Causes, Care, and Consequences*, L. D. Breslau and M. R. Haug (eds.), Springer, New York, pp. 94-113, 1983.
4. R. J. Havighurst and R. Albrecht, *Older People*, Longmans Green, New York, 1953.
5. D. R. Hoyt, M. A. Kaiser, G. R. Peters, and N. Babchuk, Life Satisfaction and Activity Theory: A Multidimensional Approach, *Journal of Gerontology, 35*:6, pp. 935-941, 1980.
6. B. Lemon, V. Bengtson, and J. Peterson, An Exploration of the Activity Theory of Aging: Activity Tapes and Life Satisfaction among In-Movers to a Retirement Community, *Journal of Gerontology, 27*:4, pp. 511-523, 1972.
7. Z. Harel, Discriminating between Survivors and Non-Survivors among Working Class Aged Living in the Community, *The Gerontologist, 19*:1, pp. 83-89, 1979.
8. V. L. Greene and D. Monahan, The Impact of Visitation on Patient Well-Being in Nursing Homes, *The Gerontologist, 22*:4, pp. 418-423, 1982.
9. P. E. Qualls, B. Justice, and R. E. Allen, Isolation and Psychosocial Functioning, *Psychological Reports, 46:*1, pp. 279-285, 1980.
10. L. J. Beckman, Effects of Social Interaction and Children's Relative Inputs on Older Women's Psychological Well Being, *Journal of Personality and Social Psychology, 41*:6, pp. 1075-1086, 1981.
11. R. Snow and L. Crapo, Emotional Bondedness, Subjective Well-Being, and Health in Elderly Medical Patients, *Journal of Gerontology, 37*:5, pp. 609-615, 1982.
12. L. J. Epstein, Depression in the Elderly, *Journal of Gerontology, 31*:3, pp. 278-282, 1976.
13. R. Murray, M. M. Huelskoetter, and D. O'Driscoll, *The Nursing Process in Later Maturity*, Prentice-Hall Inc., Englewood Cliffs, New Jersey, 1980.
14. S. M. Jourard and P. Richman, Disclosure Output and Input in College Students, *Merrill-Palmer Quarterly, 9:*1, pp. 141-148, 1963.
15. M. Worthy, A. Gary, and G. Kahn, Self-Disclosure as an Exchange Process, *Journal of Personality and Social Psychology, 13*:1, pp. 59-64, 1969.
16. S. M. Jourard, Self-Disclosure and Other-Cathexis, *Journal of Abnormal and Social Psychology, 59*:3, pp. 428-431, 1959.
17. S. M. Jourard and M. J. Landsman, Cognition, Cathexis, and the "Dyadic Effect" in Men's Self-Disclosing Behavior, *Merrill-Palmer Quarterly, 6*:2, pp. 178-186, 1960.
18. W. W. Zung, A Self-Rating Depression Scale, *Archives of General Psychiatry, 12*:1, pp. 63-70, 1965.
19. M. D. Blumenthal, Measuring Depressive Symptomatology in a General Population, *Archives of General Psychiatry, 32*, pp. 971-978, 1975.
20. J. M. Berry, M. Storandt, and A. Coyne, Age and Sex Differences in Somatic Complaints Associated with Depression, *Journal of Gerontology, 39*:4, pp. 465-467, 1984.

21. J. Steuer, L. Bank, E. J. Olsen, and F. J. Lissy, Depression, Physical Health, and Somatic Complaints in the Elderly: A Study of the Zung Self-Rating Depression Scale, *Journal of Gerontology, 35*:5, pp. 683-688, 1980.
22. L. C. Miller, J. H. Berg, and R. L. Archer, Openers: Individuals Who Elicit Intimate Self-Disclosure, *Journal of Personality and Social Psychology, 44*:6, pp. 1234-1244, 1983.
23. C. I. Cohen and H. Rajkowski, What's In a Friend? Substantive and Theoretical Issues, *The Gerontologist, 22*:3, pp. 261-266, 1982.
24. W. R. Looft and D. C. Charles, Egocentrism and Social Interaction in Young and Old Adults, *Aging and Human Development, 2,* pp. 221-228, 1971.
25. R. L. Selman and A. P. Selman, Children's Ideas About Friendship: A New Theory, *Psychology Today,* pp. 71-81, October 1979.

Section II

Health and
Social Context

Chapter 6

EMPLOYMENT, SOCIAL NETWORKS, AND HEALTH IN THE RETIREMENT YEARS

Michál E. Mor-Barak, Andrew E. Scharlach
Lourdes Birba and Jacque Sokolov

The increased interest in employment of older adults is motivated by several factors. First, the American work force is aging. The baby boom generation is getting older and is succeeded by a declining number of young people entering the work force [1]. Second, increased life expectancy rates combined with a continuing trend for early retirement amplify the economic burden of retirement on society [2]. Third, the economic reality for many older adults includes lack of sufficient income and benefits which require their continued involvement in the work force [3]. And, finally, many older adults can anticipate a prolonged and healthy aging and are interested in continuing their productive involvement in society [4].

Despite this interest in employment of older adults, the effect of continued employment after retirement on older adults' health and mental health is unclear. Studies of the relationship between retirement and health indicate that, contrary to popular belief, retirement does not necessarily adversely affect health [5-8]. At the same time, continued employment into old age generally is associated with higher morale, happiness, adjustment, and longevity [9, 10]. For example, Bossé et al. [11] examined psychological symptoms in a sample of 1,513 older men and found that retirees reported more psychological symptoms than did workers, even after controlling for physical health status. A randomized controlled study conducted by Soumerai and Avorn [12] on the impact of part-time work in a sample of retirees revealed significant positive effects of paid employment on measures of perceived health and life satisfaction. And, results of a nationally representative sample of elderly women indicated that employed women reported significantly higher levels of life satisfaction compared to members of the same cohort who were homemakers or retirees [13].

Continued employment after retirement is an activity that carries with it a number of formal and informal relationships and affiliations which potentially can provide the individual with a larger social network. However, this issue rarely has been the focus of empirical research. Studies of young and middle-aged adults have provided evidence that paid employment can have beneficial consequences for psychological well-being [14-16]. Most of the research which documented the positive effects of employment on health, focused on emotional indicators such as life satisfaction and emotional well-being and there has been very little empirical inquiry into the effects of employment on actual and perceived physical health. In addition, the mechanisms through which employment may affect perceived health were not examined. Specifically, the relationship between employment and social networks in later years needs to be explored.

The literature that deals specifically with employment as a source of social relationships has primarily focused on links between unemployment and social support in younger cohorts [17-20]. Among older cohorts, social ties may play an important role [21], particularly in light of the significant changes found to occur in the networks of elderly persons [22, 23]. Older people are also more vulnerable to life changes such as loss of a spouse, retirement, and forced relocation, situations characterized by presumed loss of social connections. Social ties, therefore, may be particularly important in sustaining the elderly's health and in decreasing their susceptibility to illness and disease [24].

Scientific investigations begun over a decade ago continue to provide evidence suggesting a positive relationship between social relationships and physical and mental health [25-29]. This effect is hypothesized to occur through several mechanisms such as providing health-related information, tangible resources, and promoting health behaviors [30]. Since research to date has established the causal relationship between social relationships and health, it follows that if a link can be identified between employment and social networks, that link may explain some of the beneficial effects of employment on the health of older adults.

This chapter focuses on three questions: 1) Does employment affect health? 2) Is the effect direct, or indirect through the effect employment may have on the individual's social network? and, 3) Which part of the network is affected by the individual's employment?

RESEARCH METHODS

Sample and Source of Data

The analysis presented in this chapter is based on data from the initial phase of Generation, a corporate sponsored geriatric clinic. Southern California Edison, a public utility company which self-insures and self-administers its employee health plans, has implemented this case managed program for its retirees. The program operates out of the company's health care centers, and includes comprehensive psychosocial and medical assessments and treatment by a multidisciplinary team. Its goals are: 1) to achieve higher quality of care by providing services that are geared toward the specific needs of elderly patients; and 2) to achieve cost savings by making more efficient use of private and public resources.

This chapter presents an analysis of data generated from comprehensive assessment questionnaires completed by participants at the time of enrollment in Generation. One hundred seventy-five questionnaires were completed by patients who were admitted to the Generation pilot program in Santa Ana, California between July and December of 1989. The average age of participants was seventy. One fourth were ages fifty-five to sixty-four, almost one half were sixty-five to seventy-four, and about one fourth were seventy-five years or older. Gender representation was almost equal, with 52 percent men and 48 percent women. Most were married (83%), Caucasian (98%), had at least some college education (69%), and had monthly incomes in the $2000-$4000 range (51%). Only 14.3 percent reported living alone.

Measures

The analytic model included the following variables: employment status, self-perceived health, social network, chronic health conditions, Activities of Daily Living (ADL), Independent Activities of Daily Living (IADL), number of hospitalizations in the past two months, number of days in bed due to physical illness in the past two months, age, gender, and education.

Employment was coded from participants' responses to the question: Were you employed or self-employed during the past twelve months? A positive response to the question, including full-time or part-time employment during the past year was coded as one = employed. A negative response was coded as zero = not employed.

The main health indicator chosen for this study was self-rated health, which was assessed by asking respondents to rate their general health from one = poor to five = excellent. The validity of the various measures of health available in the literature has long been subject for debate and empirical research. Given the importance of the health indicator in this study, a thorough consideration was given to the choice of the measure for health. The validity of self-rated health has been widely confirmed in recent literature which found significant relationships between self-health rating and mortality [31, 32]. Self-rated health has been found to correlate well with several objective indices such as number of physician visits, impairment reported in medical records, number of current medications and diagnoses, and time in hospital among non-institutionalized elderly [33]. Cross-sectional research by Maddox consistently supported the association between self-ratings and physicians' health ratings [34, 35], and self-ratings of health have been shown to be significant predictors of the need for utilizations of health care by older people [36]. Evidence from a national survey of older persons indicates that self-ratings of health were significantly related to measures of objective health status and thus were an economical means of gaining information about the health of elderly individuals [37].

A second measure of health, an "objective" measure of the number of chronic health conditions, was also included in the study as a control variable. Although not as comprehensive as the self-rated measure, it provides an objective evaluation of a very important dimension of older adults' health. This measure includes a list of fourteen conditions commonly experienced by elderly persons such as cancer, paralysis, stroke, and arthritis [38]. The score was based on the total number of health conditions endorsed by the respondent.

A composite measure of social networks, the Lubben Social Network Scale (LSNS), was used in this study. Developed specifically for older adult populations, the LSNS consists of ten items dealing with social connections with family and friends [38]. All ten items of social networks are highly intercorrelated (Cronbach Alpha = 0.70). The LSNS has been shown to be correlate significantly with another commonly used measure of social networks, the Berkman-Syme Social Network Index, and with mental health criterion variables [39]. The scale has also been shown to be a significant predictor of hospital use among elderly populations [38].

Self-care functioning was assessed using the ADL and IADL. The ADL examines the individual's ability to independently perform six personal care functions—bathing, dressing, toileting, transfer, continence, and feeding [40, 41]. The IADL assesses a person's independence in performing additional routine activities of daily living, such as shopping, food preparation, housework, laundry, telephoning, transportation, money management, and medications [42]. Both ADL and IADL record a simple dichotomous response to the question of independence or dependence in performing each specific function, and the overall score is calculated by merely summing up the number of items on which an individual was rated as independent. Scores on the ADL scale range from 0 to 6, and on the IADL from zero to eight. Higher scores indicate more independence in performing the tasks.

The three control variables were: age (in years), measured as a continuous variable; gender, a dichotomous variable, coded one for male and zero for female; and, level of education, from one = grade school to six = post graduate degree.

FINDINGS

Comparing Employed and Fully Retired Participants

Analysis indicated that 18 percent ($n = 31$) of the respondents were employed, and the rest were fully retired ($n = 144$). A series of t-tests, presented in Table 1, were performed in order to examine differences between these groups with respect to self-reported health, social network, demographic characteristics, functioning (ADL and IADL), and several health indicators (number of health problems, number of days in bed due to illness, and number of hospitalizations).

The results presented in Table 1 indicate that participants who were employed reported better health than the fully retired participants, with mean self-reported health of 2.97 and 2.50 respectively ($p < .01$). The employed participants also had larger social networks than their fully retired counterparts, with mean network score of 37.11 for the employed and 32.95 for the fully retired participants ($p < .01$). With respect to demographic characteristics, the employed group was younger (mean age = 66.2) than the fully retired (mean age = 71.5), and had a higher level of education compared to the fully retired ($p < .01$). With respect to functioning, although the difference between the groups on the IADL measure is statistically significant at the .05 level, both groups reported very few limitations—none for the employed and, on the average, 0.52 for the fully retired. The differences between the groups are not statistically significant with respect to any of the other health and functioning measures—ADL, number of health problems, number of days in bed due to illness, and number of hospitalizations over the past six months.

Three additional demographic characteristics, gender, marital status, and job classification before retirement (nominal level variables), were also examined using Chi Square tests. The results of these tests indicated that the groups were not significantly different with respect to any of these variables ($p > .05$).

Table 1. Characteristics of Employed and Fully Retired Participants
(*t*-Test Results of the Difference between Group Means)

	Employed Mean	Fully Retired Mean	*t*	prob > |*t*|
Self-reported health	2.97	2.50	−2.70	.0076**
Social network	37.11	32.95	−3.20	.0016**
Age	66.2	71.5	3.25	.0014**
Level of education	4.29	3.66	−3.75	.0002**
IADL	0.00	0.52	2.11	.03*
ADL	0.42	0.70	1.22	.22
Number of health problems	0.48	0.50	0.15	.88
Number of days in bed due to illness	0.32	0.31	−0.04	.97
Number of hospitalizations	0.61	0.74	0.53	.59

*Significant at the .05 level.
**Significant at the .01 level.

Regression Analyses: Employment, Social Network and Self-Reported Health

Given the *t*-tests results indicating significant differences in self-reported health and social networks of retirees who are employed and those who are not, the analysis proceeded to the next stage. In order to control for factors that might be related to employment, social network, and self-reported health (i.e., age, gender, education, and health problems) the study employed two regression analyses. The results of the first regression, showing the effect of employment on social networks, are presented in Table 2. They indicate that even after controlling for age, gender, education, and number of health problems, employment is significantly related to social networks ($p < .05$). Note that although the total variance explained by this regression is modest (7%) the employment variable is its main contributor since none of the other variables in the regression equation is statistically significant.

Table 3 presents the results of the second regression analysis which examines the relationship between employment, social networks, and self-reported health controlling for age, gender, education, and health problems. The results indicate that when these additional variables are entered into the regression equation the relationship between employment and self-reported health, which was statistically significant in the *t*-test (Table 1), becomes non-significant, while social network is still significantly related to self-reported health ($p < .01$). This regression equation accounts for 28 percent of the variance in self-reported health.

Thus, the results reported in the above regressions indicate that participants' employment is significantly related to social networks and, through this relationship, indirectly affects self-reported health. The next logical step, therefore, is to explore which aspects of the social network are affected by the individual's employment. This analytic process involves two stages: first, an analysis of the factor structure of the social network measure used in this study; and, second, a series of regression analyses examining the relationship between employment and each of the factors that emerge.

Factor Analysis of the Social Network Measure

Factor analysis of the LSNS detected three factors, accounting for about two-thirds of the total variance. A varimax rotation was employed to better interpret these three factors. The results are presented in Table 4. These three factors suggest that the LSNS combines three aspects of social relationships. The three dimensions are: 1) family network (frequency of contact, number individual feels "close to," number seen monthly), 2) friends network (frequency of contact, number individual feels "close to," number seen monthly); and 3) confidant relationship (has a confidant, is a confidant). Two additional items, living arrangements and "relied upon and helps others" loaded onto the family network factor,

Table 2. Regression Analysis of the Relationship between
Employment and Social Network

Dependent Variable: Social Network

Variable	Parameter Estimate	Standard Error	p
Age	−0.02	0.06	N.S.
Gender	−0.42	1.01	N.S.
Education	0.57	0.62	N.S.
Health problems	−0.43	0.40	N.S.
Employment	3.16	1.46	0.03*
Intercept	33.24	5.48	0.00**
R^2	0.07		

*Significant at the .05 level.
**Significant at the .01 level.

Table 3. Regression Analysis of the Relationship between Employment,
Social Network and Self-Reported Health

Dependent Variable: Self-Reported Health

Variable	Parameter Estimate	Standard Error	p
Age	−0.022	.010	0.03*
Gender	−0.146	0.156	N.S.
Education	−0.118	0.998	N.S.
Health problems	−0.236	0.060	0.001**
Employment	0.042	0.239	N.S.
Social network	0.040	0.013	0.003
Intercept	8.473	1.75	0.00**
R^2	0.28		

*Significant at the .05 level.
**Significant at the .01 level.

Table 4. Factor Loadings of the Social Network Scale (LSNS) Items

	Family Network	Friends Network	Confidant Relationships
Frequency of family contact	0.68	—	—
Number of family members feels "close to"	0.65	—	—
Number of family seen monthly	0.58	—	—
Living arrangements	0.48	—	—
Relied upon and helps others	0.40	—	—
Frequency of friends contact	—	0.65	—
Number of friends feels "close to"	—	0.76	—
Number of friends seen monthly	—	0.78	—
Has a confidant	—	—	0.84
Is a confidant	—	—	0.80

Note: Factor loadings <.35 have been suppressed.

suggesting that these two items are closely connected to the family dimensions of the social network.

The final step of the analysis included exploration of the relationship between employment and each of the social network factors which emerged from the factor analysis. The analysis included a series of three regressions, each with a different factor of the social network as the dependent variable. These regressions are presented in Table 5.

The analysis presented in Table 5 indicates that employment is significantly related to the friends network ($\alpha = .05$), but not to any of the other social network dimensions. An interesting pattern emerges from these regressions with respect to age and its relationship to the various aspects of the social network. Age is negatively related to the family network, but positively related to the friends network, which indicates, perhaps, that older adults may compensate for the loss of relatives (parents, spouses, siblings) by expanding the friendship network.

SUMMARY AND DISCUSSION

The study results indicate that employment in the retirement years is related to having a larger social network, and indirectly, through this relationship, to better perceived health. The analysis further explored the factor structure of the network variable and identified three factors: family network, friends network, and confidant relationships. Additional analyses revealed that of these three

Table 5. Regression Analyses of the Relationships Between Employment
and the Three Dimensions of Social Network

Dependent variable:	Family Network		Friends Network		Confidant Relationships	
Variable	Parameter Estimate	p	Parameter Estimate	p	Parameter Estimate	p
Age	−0.056	0.007**	0.084	0.001**	−0.025	N.S.
Gender	0.029	N.S.	−0.490	N.S.	0.061	N.S.
Education	0.058	N.S.	0.094	N.S.	0.168	N.S.
Health problems	−0.132	N.S.	−0.063	N.S.	−0.048	N.S.
Employment	−0.014	N.S.	1.23	0.03*	1.036	N.S.
Intercept	11.69	0.00**	0.814	0.00**	10.27	0.00**
	$R^2 = 0.07$		$R^2 = 0.10$		$R^2 = 0.03$	

*Significant at the .05 level.
**Significant at the .01 level.

dimensions, employment was positively and significantly related only to the friendship factor.

The study's major limitation is that it is cross-sectional, and therefore no conclusions can be drawn about the causal relationship between employment and health. Further, it is possible that those who are employed in the retirement years are those who are healthier rather than the other way around. There is an ongoing debate in the literature concerning this issue. Several authors [43-45] have noted the difficulty in determining whether illness, even when its onset precedes retirement, is actually causally related to retirement or is used as a convenient excuse for retirement. Although nationwide statistics on individuals retiring due to ill health are not available (except for early retirement), there is some indication that their proportion in the retiree population is relatively small [46]. For example, a New Beneficiary Survey conducted by the Social Security Administration reported that two-thirds of respondents were in good health and had no health related work limitations [47]. A study by Colsher, Dorfman, and Wallace [43] indicated that only 18 percent of 2,123 elderly individuals surveyed were retired due to ill-health. Their findings also indicated that individuals who retired for reasons other than health and those who were still working had similar lifetime history rates of specific health conditions. Similarly, in our study, the employed and the fully retired participants were not significantly different in most of the objective health and functioning measures—number of health problems, number of days in bed in the past two months due to illness, number of hospitalizations, and ADL. The only exception was in the IADL measure in which the difference between the two groups, although statistically significant, was very small. It, therefore, does not seem plausible that objective health was the reason for being employed or not being employed in the first place.

Another limitation of the study is self-selection of participants. Of the 750 Southern California Edison retirees and their dependents residing within ten miles of the Santa Ana clinic 177 decided to enroll in the program. This introduces a bias into the sample and limits the generalizability of the results.

The study's finding that social network is positively and significantly related to self-reported health is in line with the accumulating evidence that social relationships have a positive effect on an individual's health [for example, 25, 27, 48, 49]. A selection process in which more healthy and happy individuals establish a greater number of social ties than others may also account for the relationship between social networks and health [50]. However, the majority of the longitudinal research available on social networks and social support indicates a causal model in which social relationships affect subsequent well-being [49, 51-53]. It would be important nonetheless to consider both selection and causation processes in future research on employment, social networks, and health using longitudinal data.

The study's findings support the notion that employment may become an important source for enlarging an individual's friendship network in later life. Of the three factors that emerged as a result of the factor analysis—the family network, friends network, and confidant relationships—the friends network was the one which was significantly related to employment. The importance of co-workers in social networks is demonstrated by the work of various researchers [54-56]. Fischer found that work was the most important source of non-kin relationships among persons who were employed [55]. Furthermore, employed persons reported a greater number of contacts with non-kin than did those who were not employed. Thus, employment apparently provides opportunities to meet and develop relationships with others, opportunities which may be lacking for those who are fully retired.

This study highlights the potential positive effects of employment in the retirement years for social networks and health. Longitudinal research is needed to help clarify the causal relationships between employment social networks and health in the retirement years.

PRACTICE AND POLICY IMPLICATIONS

The trend toward early retirement, coupled with the diminishing numbers of youth entering the labor market as a result of lower post baby-boom birth rates, presents American industry with an impending shortage of available workers [1]. Concurrently, many older adults can anticipate a prolonged and healthy aging and would welcome the opportunity for part-time flexible jobs. Such continued activity corresponds to a wish to remain contributing members of society as well as to supplement their income [57, 58]. The present study indicates that, in addition to its financial benefits to individuals and society, employment is associated with better social networks and better health of older adults.

Although we cannot draw any conclusions about causal relationships based on this cross-sectional data, the results lead to some suggested implications for practice and policy. Practice implications include a recommendation for social and health care providers who serve older persons to become more active in helping their clients find meaningful jobs, by developing linkages with employment agencies and informing older adults of employment opportunities in their communities. Interventions such as these may be particularly important through the next several decades, as the population of older Americans rapidly increases. Providing flexible, meaningful employment opportunities could help to make up for some of the losses in social as well as economic resources experienced by most older adults.

The involvement of social workers and other professionals in community efforts to create additional job opportunities for older adults is critical. Lack of success due to an economic labor market demand deficiency may create feelings of depression, isolation, and job search discouragement in older adults seeking employment [59]. Greater public resources may need to be targeted toward assisting older adults in gaining meaningful employment. Expanded job training and public service job programs are important points for advocacy in this regard. Studies which demonstrate the benefits of hiring older workers are needed. Expanding programs for participating in group job placement (such as "job clubs") and retaining activities are also important. Individual counseling can be beneficial, particularly to older adults who have been out of the work force or out of the job search process for a long time, or for those experiencing age discrimination.

For most Americans, retirement has become an acceptable, even welcome part of life. Retirement counselors and educators need to be aware that certain retiree groups (e.g., those who retire because of health) may need more information about health care than do other groups. Information concerning health care programs can be targeted specifically to the needs of the elderly. For those older individuals who want or need to work, however, obstacles still exist. Barriers that keep people from participating in the paid labor force serve to limit the nation's overall productivity, and limit individuals' choices and options. For example, complaints of age discrimination in employment filed with state and federal agencies more than doubled between 1981 and 1987. Of those complaints filed with the Equal Employment Opportunity Commission (EEOC), more than half involved loss of employment [60]. Efforts may be directed towards advocacy to promote the hiring of older workers and to combat ageism [61]. Practices such as mandatory retirement, refusal to hire middle-aged individuals, and preferences for promoting younger workers create barriers to employment of older adults and constitute age discrimination. A congressional statute, the Age Discrimination in Employment Act (ADEA) extends the concept of discrimination to age and prohibits most of these age/work practices [62]. Emotional support and legal aid can be helpful services to older adults who are victims of age discrimination.

The relationship between retirement and health is a complex combination of a number of factors. Financial incentives as well as psychological and social functions of work play roles in work-retirement decisions. Given the study's findings indicating the potential positive relationship between employment, social networks, and health of older adults, attempts at intervention may prolong older adults' participation in the work force and improve their quality of life.

REFERENCES

1. W. B. Johnson and A. E. Packer, *Workforce 2000: Work and Workers for the 21st Century*, Hudson Institute, Indianapolis, Indiana, 1987.
2. R. L. Clark, The Future of Work and Retirement, *Research on Aging, 10*:2, pp. 169-193, 1988.
3. M. I. Howard, Employment of Retired-Worker Women, *Social Security Bulletin, 49*:3, pp. 4-18, 1986.
4. M. D. Hayward, W. R. Grady, and S. D. McLaughlin, Recent Changes in Mortality and Labor Force Behavior among Older Americans: Consequences for Nonworking Life Expectancy, *Journal of Gerontology, 43*:6, pp. S194-199, 1988.
5. D. J. Ekerdt, Why the Notion Persists that Retirement Harms Health, *The Gerontologist, 27*:4, pp. 454-457, 1987.
6. D. J. Ekerdt, L. Baden, R. Bossé, and E. Dibbs, The Effects of Retirement on Physical Health, *American Journal of Public Health, 73*, pp. 779-783, 1983.
7. S. V. Kasl, The Impact of Retirement, in *Current Concerns in Occupational Stress*, C. L. Cooper and R. Payne (eds.), John Wiley, New York, 1980.
8. E. B. Palmore, B. M. Burchett, G. G. Fillbaum, L. K. George, and L. M. Wallman, *Retirement: Causes and Consequences*, Springer, New York, 1985.
9. K. A. Conner, L. T. Dorfman, and J. B. Tompkins, Life Satisfaction of Retired Professors: The Contribution of Work, Health, Income, and Length of Retirement, *Educational Gerontology, 11*, pp. 337-347, 1985.
10. E. B. Palmore and V. Stone, Predictors of Longevity: A Follow-Up of the Aged in Chapel Hill, *The Gerontologist, 13*, pp. 88-90, 1973.
11. R. Bossé, C. M. Aldwin, M. R. Levenson, and D. J. Ekerdt, Mental Health Differences among Retirees and Workers: Findings from the Normative Aging Study, *Psychology and Aging, 2*:4, pp. 383-389, 1987.
12. S. B. Soumerai and J. Avorn, Perceived Health, Life Satisfaction, and Activity in Urban Elderly: A Controlled Study of the Impact of Part-Time Work, *Journal of Gerontology, 38*, pp. 356-362, 1983.
13. C. C. Riddick, Life Satisfaction for Older Female Homemakers, Retirees, and Workers, *Research on Aging, 7*:3, pp. 383-393, 1985.
14. S. Cobb and S. V. Kasl, *Termination: The Consequences of Job Loss*, U.S. Department of Health, Education and Welfare, HEW (NIOSH) Publication, No. 77-224, Washington, D.C., U.S. Government Printing Office, 1977.

15. J. Veroff, E. Douvan, and R. Kulka, *The Inner American: A Self-Portrait from 1957 to 1976*, Basic Books, New York, 1981.
16. P. Warr and G. Parry, Depressed Mood in Working-Class Mothers With and Without Paid Employment, *Social Psychiatry, 1*:4, pp. 161-165, 1982.
17. S. Gore, The Effect of Social Support in Moderating the Health Consequences of Unemployment, *Journal of Health and Social Behavior, 19*, pp. 157-165, 1978.
18. L. I. Pearlin, E. G. Menaghan, M. A. Liberman, and J. T. Mullan, The Stress Process, *Journal of Health and Social Behavior, 22*, pp. 337-356, 1981.
19. S. K. Rathcliff and J. Bogdan, Unemployed Women: When "Social Support" is Not Supportive, *Social Problems, 35*:1, pp. 54-63, 1988.
20. T. Aubry, B. Tefft, and N. Kingsbury, Behavioral and Psychological Consequences of Unemployment in Blue Collar Couples, *Journal of Community Psychology, 18*(April), pp. 99-109, 1990.
21. J. Treas, Family Support Systems for the Aged, Some Social and Demographic Considerations, *The Gerontologist, 17*:6, pp. 486-491, 1977.
22. T. T. H. Wan, *Stressful Life Events, Social Support Network and Gerontological Health*, D.C. Health, Lexington, Massachusetts, 1982.
23. R. L. Kahn, Aging and Social Support, in *Aging From Birth to Death*, M. W. Riley (ed.), Westview Press, Boulder, Colorado, 1979.
24. M. Minkler and M. Pilisuk, *Social Support and Health: Implications for Graying America,* paper presented to the 110th Annual Meeting of the American Public Health Association, Montreal, Canada, 1982.
25. L. Berkman and S. L. Syme, Social Networks, Host Resistance, and Mortality: A Nine-Year Follow-Up Study of Alameda County Residents, *American Journal of Epidemiology, 109*:2, pp. 186-204, 1979.
26. W. E. Broadhead, B. H. Kaplan, J. A. James, E. H. Wagner, V. J. Schoenbach, et al. The Epidemiologic Evidence for a Relationship between Social Support and Health, *American Journal of Epidemiology, 117*:5, pp. 521-537, 1983.
27. J. S. House, C. Robbins, and H. Metzner, The Association of Social Relationships and Activities with Mortality: Prospective Evidence from the Tecumseh Community Health Study, *American Journal of Epidemiology, 116*, pp. 123-140, 1982.
28. M. E. Mor-Barak, L. S. Miller, and L. S. Syme, Social Networks, Life Events and Health of the Poor Frail Elderly: A Longitudinal Study of the Buffering versus the Direct Effect, *Family and Community Health, 14*:2, pp. 1-3, 1991.
29. V. J. Schoenbach, B. H. Kaplan, D. G. Kleinbaoum, and D. G. Grekman, *Social Ties and Mortality,* paper presented at the Annual Meeting of the American Public Health Association, Dallas, Texas, 1983.
30. S. Cohen, Psychosocial Models of the Role of Social Support in the Etiology of Physical Disease, *Health Psychology, 7*:3, pp. 269-297, 1988.
31. G. A. Kaplan and T. Camacho, Perceived Health and Mortality: A Nine-Year Follow-Up of the Human Population Laboratory Cohort, *American Journal of Epidemiology, 117*:3, pp. 292-304, 1983.
32. J. M. Mossey and E. Shapiro, Self-Rated Health: A Predictor of Mortality among the Elderly, *American Journal of Public Health, 72*:8, pp. 800-808, 1982.

33. B. S. Linn and M. W. Linn, Objective and Self-Assessed Health in the Old and Very Old, *Social Science and Medicine, 14A*, pp. 311-315, 1980.
34. G. L. Maddox and E. B. Douglas, Self-Assessment of Health: A Longitudinal Study of Elderly Subjects, *Journal of Health and Social Behavior, 14*, pp. 87-93, 1973.
35. G. L. Maddox, Self Assessment of Health Status: A Longitudinal Study of Selected Elderly Subjects, *Journal of Chronic Disease, 17*, pp. 449-460, 1964.
36. M. Markides, Self-Rated Health, *Research on Aging, 1*:1, pp. 98-112, 1979.
37. K. F. Ferraro, Self-Ratings of Health among the Old and the Old-Old, *Journal of Health and Social Behavior, 21*, pp. 377-383, 1980.
38. J. E. Lubben, Assessing Social Networks among Elderly Populations, *Journal of Family and Community Health, 11*, pp. 42-52, 1988.
39. J. E. Lubben, P. G. Weiler, and I. Chi, Health Practices of the Elderly Poor, *American Journal of Public Health, 74*:4, pp. 1-4, 1989.
40. S. Katz and C. A. Akpom, A Measure of Primary Sociobiological Functions, *International Journal of Health Services, 6*, pp. 493-507, 1976.
41. S. Katz, T. D. Downs, H. R. Cash, and R. C. Grotz, Progress in Development of the Index of ADL, *The Gerontologist, 10*, pp. 20-30, 1970.
42. M. P. Lawton and E. M. Brody, Assessment of Older People: Self Maintenance and Instrumental Activities of Daily Living, *The Gerontologist, 9*, pp. 176-186, 1969.
43. P. L. Colsher, L. T. Dorfman, and R. B. Wallace, Specific Health Conditions and Work-Retirement Status among the Elderly, *Journal of Applied Gerontology, 7*:4, pp. 485-503, 1988.
44. R. J. Myers, Why do People Retire Early? *Social Security Bulletin, 45*, pp. 10-14, 1982.
45. E. R. Kingson, The Health of Very Early Retirees, *Social Security Bulletin, 45*, pp. 3-9, 1982.
46. J. M. Mitchell and K. H. Anderson, Mental Health and the Labor Force Participation of Older Workers, *Inquiry, 26*, pp. 262-271, 1989.
47. M. Packard, Health Status of New Retired-Worker Beneficiaries: Findings from the New Beneficiary Survey, *Social Security Bulletin, 48*:2, pp. 5-16, 1985.
48. D. G. Blazer, Social Support and Mortality in an Elderly Community Population, *American Journal of Epidemiology, 115*, pp. 684-694, 1982.
49. M. E. Mor-Barak and L. S. Miller, A Longitudinal Study of the Causal Relationship between Social Networks and Health of the Poor Frail Elderly, *Journal of Applied Gerontology, 10*:2, pp. 293-310, 1991.
50. D. Dooley, Causal Inference in the Study of Social Support, in *Social Support and Health*, S. Cohen and S. L. Syme (eds.), Academic Press, New York, 1985.
51. C. J. Holahan and R. H. Moos, Social Support and Psychological Distress: A Longitudinal Analysis, *Journal of Abnormal Psychology, 90*, pp. 365-370, 1984.
52. R. J. Turner, Social Support as a Contingency in Psychological Well-Being, *Journal of Health and Social Behavior, 22*, pp. 357-367, 1981.
53. P. A. Thoits, Explaining Distributions of Psychological Vulnerability: Lack of Social Support in the Face of Life Stress, *Social Forces, 63*, pp. 453-481, 1984.
54. A. H. McFarlane, D. A. Neale, R. G. Roy, and D. L. Streiner, Methodological Issues in Developing a Scale to Measure Social Support, *Schizophrenia Bulletin, 7*, pp. 90-100, 1981.

55. C. S. Fischer, *To Dwell Among Friends: Personal Networks in Town and City*, University of Chicago Press, Chicago, Illinois, 1982.
56. C. S. Fischer and S. J. Oliker, A Research Note on Friendship, Gender and the Life-Cycle, *Social Forces, 62*:1, pp. 124-133, 1983.
57. B. Bourne, Effects of Aging on Work Satisfaction, Performance and Motivation, *Aging and Work, 5*, pp. 37-47, 1982.
58. J. Sonnenfeld, Continued Work Contributions in Late Career, in *Fourteen Steps in Managing an Aging Work Force*, H. Dennis (ed.), Lexington Books, Massachusetts, pp. 191-211, 1988.
59. J. Rife and K. Kilty, Job Search Discouragement and the Older Worker: Implications for Social Work Practice, *Journal of Applied Social Sciences, 14*:1, pp. 71-94, 1989-90.
60. American Association of Retired Persons (AARP), *Aging in America: Dignity or Despair?* Washington, D.C., 1988.
61. M. E. Mor-Barak and M. Tynan, Older Workers and the Work Place: A New Challenge for Occupational Social Work, *Social Work* (in press), 1992.
62. M. L. Levine, Age Discrimination: The Law and its Underlying Policy, in *Fourteen Steps in Managing an Aging Work Force*, H. Dennis (ed.), Lexington Books, Massachusetts, pp. 25-38, 1988.

Chapter 7

RURAL VERSUS URBAN DIFFERENCES IN HEALTH DEPENDENCE AMONG THE ELDERLY POPULATION

John A. Krout

The level and determinants of health status among elderly people have received considerable attention in the gerontological literature. Research has also focused on variations in health status for the elderly population based on factors such as sex, income, race, and marital status. Another factor that has been given substantially less attention in health research has been that of community type or, more specifically, rural versus urban differences. A number of studies of elderly rural residents indicate that they experience the same kind of chronic health problems as the general elderly population including difficulties with: arthritis, blood pressure, respiratory system, heart, digestive track, sight, and hearing [1, 2].

As for rural versus urban differences in the level of physical health status, there are reasons to expect both better or worse health for the rural aged. On the one hand, it can be argued that rural areas have cleaner air, are less congested, and have a slower pace than urban areas. On the other hand, it can be argued that the lower incomes of rural elderly people and less adequate medical services would contribute negatively to their health as would their supposedly less adequate housing, transportation, and recreational opportunities [3, 4]. Without addressing the question of why such differences exist, the majority of research on reported ailments and impairments indicates the health status of the rural elderly population is not as good as their urban counterparts.

In fact, one comprehensive review of the literature on rural versus urban health differences has stated:

No matter what measurement of health status is used—self-assessment by the elderly individual of health as excellent, good, fair, or poor; reports of ailments; reports of mobility limitations; use of health aids or prescription drugs; number of days hospitalized; or any combination of these—the results are always the same: the rural elderly are in relatively poor health [5, p. 94].

For example, Youmans' comparison of aged sixty and over Kentucky men living in a rural county and a metropolitan area revealed the rural residents were more likely to report ailments (72% vs. 57%) and that physical impairments kept them from doing usual activities sometime in the last five years (63% vs. 45%) [3]. He reported similar rural versus urban differences in a later study as well [6]. Rural disadvantagement is also reported by Nelson, Kivett and Scott, Paringer et al., and Schooler [1, 7-9].

Several studies examining national or regional health statistics have also reported higher incidence of health problems among the rural elderly population. For example, McCoy and Brown, in an analysis of Social Security Administration data on low-income elderly people, reported that chronic disorders and impairments were more prevalent among rural than urban residents even when sex, age, and race were statistically controlled [10]. Focusing on a different elderly population, Dahlstein and Shank found that rural nursing home patients had a greater average number of chronic diseases than is reported nationally [11].

An examination of national data from the early 1960s led Ellenbcgen to conclude that the health status of rural elderly people compared unfavorably to the urban on a number of indicators including: incidence of acute conditions, selected chronic conditions and impairments, and incidences of injuries or disability [12]. Moreover, Palmore, using more recent data from the National Center on Health Statistics, concluded that rural elders have more sickness and disability that their urban counterparts [13]. Burkhardt et al. also reported that an analysis of 1975 vital and health statistics revealed the rural elderly population experienced more restricted mobility than the urban in all regions of the country with the largest community size differences in the South [14]. Palmore presented national health statistics data that further revealed elderly farm dwellers to have slightly lower rates of impairment than the nonmetropolitan nonfarm elderly [13].

Given such a preponderance of research findings it would seem reasonable to assert that the rural elderly population is in fact less healthy. However, caution is suggested in accepting such a generalization without qualification. First, in most of the studies reviewed above, statistical tests are not used to determine the magnitude of the differences. That is, the findings reported may not reflect a large enough difference to be considered significant. The question that should be asked is whether or not the reported differences are large enough to justify a conclusion that rural elderly people are less healthy. In addition, multivariate analyses are particularly lacking and appropriate controls are often not used. The impact of community type, apart from differences in basic population characteristics, is often not demonstrated. Second, as is the case in many studies of the rural versus urban elderly population, the definition of rural and urban is not always stated.

For example, Palmore's report distinguished between the "rural nonfarm" and "farm" elderly and a category labeled "all residences" [13]. The reader is not told what distinguishes rural farm and nonfarm. Let us assume that rural nonfarm refers to people living in places of less than 2,500 but not on farms. A close look at the data presented by Palmore shows larger differences between rural-nonfarm and farm than between rural nonfarm and the all residence category. For some health indicators rural nonfarm elderly people appear less healthy than the farm, for others they appear more healthy. No data on the statistical significance of the differences are given.

Finally, there are studies that do not find significant rural versus urban differences in the elderly person's health status. A detailed examination of national health statistics by staff members of the Urban Institute concluded that place of residence in general is not associated with significant differences in health status [8]. This conclusion is based on a review of data on a number of health status indicators for elderly people: mortality rates, incidence of acute illness, incidence of chronic illness, number of restricted activity days and days of bed disability, and self-assessed health. These authors find some differences based on residence, but state they are usually neither large nor consistent. The major exception was based on disability days. Here it was discovered that male farm dwellers experienced the greatest number of restricted activity days. They also found some variation by geographic region with white elderly males living in the Southeast and mining areas reporting the highest chronic illness rate for that sub-group.

These drawbacks and inconsistent findings suggest that more systematic research needs to be carried out before the magnitude and nature of rural versus urban health status differences are clearly demonstrated. Lassey and Lassey observed that rural versus urban differences in health status may result from intervening factors such as lower income and health risks and poor health care associated with it [15]. Paringer et al. argue that more multivariate research needs to be carried out, the causal direction of variables needs to be specified, and a much greater emphasis needs to be placed on longitudinal studies [8].

This chapter presents an analysis of data on the health dependency of elderly people living in a continuum of community types that addresses several of the concerns noted above. The data allow a rural versus urban comparison and are analyzed using both bivariate and multivariate statistics. It should be pointed out that the study is largely exploratory and is not designed to test any specific hypotheses concerning variation in the level or nature of health status for rural versus urban dwellers.

METHODOLOGY

Data for this study were collected via personal interviews with a random sample of 600 community dwelling individuals aged sixty-five years and over residing in western New York. These persons lived in a continuum of community settings ranging from farm areas to the central city of a metropolitan area of 1.6 million inhabitants. The distribution of the sample across residence categories is as follows: nonmetropolitan rural (less than 2,500), 26 percent; nonmetropolitan urban (more than 2,500), 24 percent; metropolitan noncentral city, 21 percent; and metropolitan central city, 29 percent.

The residential designations noted above were used to improve upon the normative practice of simply categorizing residence as rural or urban. This dichotomy ignores the fact that rural/urban is more realistically a continuum. Traditionally, the term rural has been used to designate places of less than 2,500 and the term urban has then been applied to anything else. This means small villages and giant central cities are subsumed under the same heading. In addition, since the Census Bureau adopted the metropolitan/nonmetropolitan classification, these terms have been used synonymously with urban/rural, thereby creating further impreciseness in the analysis of size of place differences. The use of metropolitan versus nonmetropolitan was incorporated along with size of place because metropolitan status is a rough indicator of the proximity of a place to the complex social, economic, and organization entity that is the modern metropolis. A place of say 10,000 to 20,000 people within a metropolitan county more than likely will be much closer to the complex infrastructure (service, transportation, etc.) of the "city" than a place of similar size in a sparsely populated area.

Trained research assistants conducted structured one-hour interviews to collect information from this sample. The overall response rate was 78 percent, with the nonmetropolitan county rate of 87 percent considerably higher than the metropolitan county rate of 71 percent. Contingency table analysis is used to uncover the bivariate relationship between community type and the variables used in this analysis. Multiple-regression analysis is used to determine if and how other variables affect the relationship between community type and health dependency. In this analysis, the community type variable is entered into the equation after all the other variables.

Sample

Data in Table 1 show the sociodemographic characteristics of participants. The sample is 57 percent female, 92 percent white, and 7 percent black. The median age is 72.8 with 36 percent aged sixty-five to sixty-nine, 30 percent aged seventy to seventy-four, 19 percent aged seventy-five to seventy-nine, and 15 percent aged eighty and over. Two-thirds of the sample live with another individual (80% of

Table 1. Selected Background Characteristics of Elderly Respondents for Total Sample and by Community Type (N = 600)[a]

Characteristic	Total Sample	Community Type				Chi Square	Significance
		nmr	nmu	mncc	mcc		
Sex							
Male	43.1	50.0	39.9	51.6	33.3		
Female	56.9	50.0	60.1	48.4	66.7	14.11	.003
Age							
65–69	36.2	37.8	35.4	31.7	38.5		
70–74	30.0	31.4	30.6	24.6	32.2		
75–79	18.7	16.7	19.4	22.2	17.2		
80 and over	15.2	14.1	14.6	21.4	12.1	8.63	.472
Race							
White	92.5	99.4	100.0	92.9	79.9		
Black	7.5	0.6	0.0	7.1	20.1	62.01	.000
Living Arrangement							
Live alone	34.8	28.8	29.9	38.1	42.0		
Live with others	65.2	71.2	70.1	61.9	58.0	8.51	.037
Marital Status							
Married	52.8	61.3	55.9	50.8	44.3		
Widowed	47.2	38.7	44.1	49.2	55.7	10.36	.016
Annual Household Income							
Less than $7,500	30.0	24.1	28.9	24.4	38.8		
$7,500–9,999	20.0	21.4	18.4	21.1	20.4		
$10,000–14,999	25.0	29.7	26.3	22.0	22.4		
$15,000 or more	25.0	24.8	26.3	32.5	18.4	15.00	.091
Education							
8 years or less	30.8	25.0	31.9	30.2	35.6		
9–11 years	26.5	27.6	22.2	24.6	30.5		
12 years	23.3	24.4	24.3	24.6	20.1		
13 years or more	19.5	23.1	21.5	20.6	13.8	10.66	.300
Home Ownership							
Own	80.1	84.6	78.9	81.0	76.4		
Rent	19.9	15.4	21.1	19.0	23.5	12.15	.059
Length of Residence in Community							
1–25 years	15.0	19.2	11.1	26.2	3.4		
26–50 years	33.5	37.8	27.1	39.7	33.3		
51–70 years	32.8	25.0	38.9	23.0	42.0		
71 or more years	18.7	17.9	22.9	11.1	21.0	53.15	.000
Length of Residence at Present Address							
1–15 years	26.3	25.0	25.0	31.0	25.3		
16–30 years	30.8	29.5	29.9	32.5	31.6		
31–45 years	29.3	28.8	29.9	23.8	33.3		
46 or more years	13.5	16.7	15.3	12.7	9.8	7.22	.614

[a] All data in percents.

these with a spouse), 53 percent are married, and 37 percent widowed. The sample has a mean 11.1 years of education with 57 percent having less than a complete high school education, 23 percent a high school education, and 9 percent with post-high school education. A wide range of household income levels is reported by the respondents: 30 percent less than $7,500, 20 percent in the $7,500 to $9,999 category, 25 percent in the $10,000 to $14,999 range, and 25 percent in the $15,000 and over range. Four-fifths of the sample own their own homes. A fairly high degree of residential stability is shown by the sample with a mean of fifty years lived in the community and 28.5 lived at the present address.

It is difficult to demonstrate with exactness how closely this sample approximates the national "average" in terms of background characteristics and thus how comfortable we can be in generalizing the results of the study. However, it would appear that in many respects the sample used in this research does match the national demographic profile of the elderly population. Many of the differences may largely be a result of the fact that the sample contains a higher percentage of nonmetropolitan elders than is found for the nation as a whole.

For example, while 41 percent of those fifty-six years and over had finished high school nationally as of 1979, 39 percent of this sample has done so [16]. This sample has a slightly smaller percentage of women than is true for the over sixty-five population in the country as a whole in 1980 (57% versus 59%, respectively), and a smaller proportion of nonwhites nationally (7% versus 9.4%) as of 1979 [16, 17]. The age distribution of the sample studied here also differs somewhat from that of the nation's elderly population in that the sample has a smaller percentage over eighty—possibly because of differences in the sex ratio.

In addition, the sample is slightly less likely to be married (53% versus a national average of 59%) and concomitantly more likely to live alone [17]. This sample reports lower household incomes than the national average. While one-third of the families headed by an individual aged sixty-five or over report household incomes of more than $15,000 nationally, only 25 percent of this sample reports that amount [17]. Yet the sample is more likely to own their own homes (80% versus 74%) [16].

Table 1 also presents data on demographic characteristics broken down by community type. Statistically significant differences are found for sex, race, marital status, living arrangement, and length of residence in the community. The elderly respondents in the central city and nonmetropolitan urban places are more likely to be female (67% and 60%, respectively). Metropolitan (central city and noncentral city) respondents are more likely to live alone (42% and 38%, respectively), be unmarried (56% and 49%, respectively), and are much more likely to be nonwhite. In fact, 20 percent of the central city sample and 7 percent of the metropolitan noncentral city is nonwhite. Finally, those elderly people living in the central city and nonmetropolitan urban places have lived there six and five years more than the mean for the total sample.

Instrument and Analysis

The protocol used in the present study consisted of twenty-three pages and 197 precoded items specific to the respondents' demographic characteristics, proximity and contact with informal networks, health dependency, ability to carry out routine activities of daily living, community living skills, and awareness and use of service programs for elderly people. Health dependency of elderly respondents is operationalized in a manner similar to that adopted by Branch [18]. It is an index composed of the following criterion measures:

1. twelve or more physician contacts over the last twelve months;
2. thirty-one or more days of hospitalization;
3. restricted at home for one month or more;
4. overnight or longer admission to a nursing home;
5. having received nursing services at home;
6. having received homemaker services;
7. having meals delivered at home;
8. use of a walker; and
9. use of a wheelchair.

From this cluster of criterion measures, a health dependency index score was obtained for each of the elders surveyed, the rationale being that those who satisfy one or more of the criteria listed are more care dependent than those who satisfy none. Respondents having used none of the services or supportive devices received a care dependency score of zero, while those indicating that they had used or are using all of them received a score of nine. Thus, the theoretical score range obtainable for the index was from zero (no dependency) to nine (maximum dependency). Elderly respondents identified as having used none of the services or devices (index equals zero) were categorized as "self-sufficient," those having used only one were characterized as "slightly dependent," while those among the respondents who reported that they had used two or more health care or support services were described as "care dependent." Needless to say, the criterion of an index score of two or more as the threshold value for the operational definition of a health care dependent elder is somewhat arbitrary.

The measurement and coding of the independent variables used in this research are shown in Table 2. These include basic sociodemographic variables that are often viewed as predisposing or enabling factors in studies of service utilization [19, 20]. In addition, a variable on amount of contact with an elder's first-mentioned child is included as an indicator of informal support. The number of services each respondent is aware of is also included in the analysis to take into account the degree of familiarity with the formal service network. Service awareness among elderly people has been found to be strongly related to service utilization [21].

Table 2. Categories and Coding of Variables Used in Multiple-Regression Analysis

Variable	Measurement	Coding
Sex	Dummy variable	0 = male 1 = female
Race	Dummy variable	0 = white 1 = nonwhite
Marital Status	Dummy variable	0 = married 1 = not married
Home Ownership	Dummy variable	0 = yes 1 = no
Car Ownership	Dummy variable	0 = yes 1 = no
Living Arrangement	Dummy variable	0 = live with someone 1 = live alone
Annual Household Income	Ordinal variable	1 = less than $7,500 2 = $7,500–$9,999 3 = $10,000–$14,999 4 = $15,000 and up
In-Person Contact with First Mentioned Child	Ordinal variable	1 = everyday 2 = several times a week 3 = few times a month 4 = once a month or less
Health Dependency[a]	Ordinal variable	0 = uses no services or devices 1 = uses one service or device 2 = uses two or more services or devices
Community Type	Ordinal variable	1 = nonmetropolitan less than 2,500 2 = nonmetropolitan greater than 2,500 3 = metropolitan outside central city 4 = metropolitan central city
Age	Interval = age in years	
Education	Interval = number of years in school	
Service Awareness	Interval = number of services known	
Length of Residence	Interval = number of years lived in community	

a Based on index of nine criterion measures [18].

FINDINGS

Using the criterion defined above, three-quarters (74.7%) of the discussed sample were classified as self-sufficient, 17.7 percent qualified as slightly dependent, and only 7.7 percent dependent. Data presented in Table 3 show the bivariate relationship between health dependence and a number of independent variables including community type. Statistically significant differences are found for five variables. Health dependence is greater for those elders who are older, nonwhite, not married, and report lower incomes. Although no linear relationship is evidenced between size of community and health status, elderly persons residing in nonmetropolitan places are *less* likely to be classified as dependent than those living in metropolitan communities. In fact, nonmetropolitan urban elderly residents appear to be considerably more healthy than their more rural and more urban counterparts.

The impact of other independent variables on the observed bivariate relationship between community size and health dependency can be determined through a multiple-regression analysis. Recall that elders who were white, married, younger, and wealthier were more likely to be classified as being self-sufficient. It is known that elderly people in rural areas in general are more likely to be male, white, or married [22]. In fact, data previously reviewed in this chapter show a significant relationship between community type and race and marital status. The more urban the place, the greater the percentage of elderly residents who are nonwhite and the smaller the percentage who are married or male. No age association with residence was found, but metropolitan central city elders were most likely to report incomes of less than $7,500. On the other hand, there is no convincing body of literature that suggests significant rural versus urban elderly age differences and considerable evidence to suggest a rural income disadvantage [22].

The results of the multiple-regression analysis are shown in Table 4. Only three of the independent variables have significant betas (age, car ownership, and income). Health dependency is greater for those who are older, report lower incomes, and do not own a car. Thus, the rural versus urban difference observed in the bivariate case is not found when independent variables are controlled for.

Because the health dependency measure can be criticized for confounding health status with health service availability and use, community type differences on self-assessed health are reported in Table 5. Significant residence differences are not observed. Bivariate differences for this health measure are found for race, income, education, home ownership, and length of residence. More positive self-assessments of health are reported for elderly persons who are: white, better educated, wealthier, and longer term residents of their communities. A similar relationship with health dependence was found for two of these variables in Table 3 (race and income). A multiple-regression analysis similar to the one performed for health dependency, but not reported in this chapter, does not show a significant impact of residence on self-assessed health.

Table 3. Health Dependency Score for Selected Independent Variables (N = 600)[a]

Characteristic	Health Dependency Score			Chi Square	Significance
	0	1	2+		
Sex					
Male	77.9	15.5	6.6		
Female	72.1	19.4	8.5	2.59	.274
Age					
65–69	82.0	13.8	4.1		
70–74	77.8	16.7	5.6		
75–79	70.5	17.9	11.6		
80 and over	56.0	28.6	15.4	28.22	.0001
Race					
White	75.3	17.9	6.9		
Other	66.7	15.6	17.8	7.00	.030
Living Arrangement					
Live alone	70.3	19.6	10.0		
Live with other	77.0	16.6	6.4	3.87	.144
Marital Status					
Married	79.4	15.8	4.7		
Not married	69.1	19.8	11.0	11.04	.004
Annual Household Income					
Less than $7,500	65.6	21.7	12.7		
$7,500–9,999	78.0	13.8	8.3		
$10,000–14,999	73.1	19.4	7.5		
$15,000 or more	82.8	14.9	2.2	16.44	.012
Education					
8 years or less	74.1	14.1	11.9		
9–11 years	74.2	18.2	7.5		
12 years	77.0	18.7	4.3		
13 years or more	73.5	21.4	5.1	9.85	.131
Home Ownership					
Own	76.0	16.7	7.3		
Rent	68.9	21.8	9.2	2.53	.282
Length of Residence in Community					
1–25 years	70.0	21.1	8.9		
26–50 years	75.1	15.9	9.0		
51–70 years	78.7	16.2	5.1		
71 or more years	70.5	20.5	8.9	8.19	.225
Community Type					
nmr	72.4	19.9	7.7		
nmu	84.0	12.5	3.5		
mncc	66.7	23.8	9.5		
mcc	74.7	15.5	9.8	13.50	.036

[a] All data in percents.

Table 4. Multiple Regression Showing the Relationship
between the Health Dependency Score and
Selected Independent Variables

Independent Variable	Beta (N = 600)
Age	.205*
Car Ownership	.109*
Annual Household Income	-.065*
Race	.049
Child Contact	.019
Education	.014
Length of Residence in Community	-.015
Service Awareness	.032
Home Ownership	-.012
Marital Status	.027
Living Arrangement	.028
Sex	.010
Community Type	-.012
R	.284
R^2	.080

* Significant at the .05 level.

DISCUSSION

As noted earlier in this chapter, the majority but not entirety of research on rural versus urban elderly health differences has found a rural health disadvantage. The data reported here do not support this generalization, but rather stand as evidence for the minority position that the direct effect of community size as a determinant of health status or dependence among the elderly population has not clearly been established. In fact, the nonmetropolitan elders in this sample overall report a *lower* degree of health dependence than the metropolitan, the opposite of what many other studies have noted. Two variables traditionally identified as predictors of health (older age and lower incomes) as well as car ownership (perhaps both a cause and effect) are the only correlates of health dependency uncovered in this research.

A closer consideration of these findings provides further support for the argument that the bulk of existing research needs to be viewed more critically. The four-fold community type typology reveals considerable differences within as well as between the nonmetropolitan and metropolitan categories. Overall,

Table 5. Self-Assessed Health for Selected Independent Variables (N = 600)[a]

	Self-Assessed Health				Chi	
Independent Variable	Poor	Fair	Good	Excellent	Square	Significance
Community Type						
Nonmetropolitan rural	4.5	28.8	44.9	21.8		
Nonmetropolitan urban	5.6	32.2	46.2	16.1		
Metropolitan suburban	3.2	23.0	50.8	23.0		
Metropolitan central city	8.1	25.0	45.9	20.9	8.74	.462
Sex						
Male	3.1	26.4	49.2	21.3		
Female	7.4	28.1	44.7	19.8	5.85	.119
Age						
65–69 years	3.7	27.2	48.8	20.3		
70–74 years	3.9	28.1	43.8	24.2		
75–79 years	7.2	26.1	49.5	17.1		
80 and over years	11.0	27.5	44.0	17.6	10.76	.292
Race						
White	4.4	27.4	47.0	21.2		
Other	20.0	26.7	42.2	11.1	20.68	.000
Living Arrangement						
Live alone	7.7	23.7	46.9	21.7		
Live with another	4.4	29.2	46.7	19.7	4.57	.206
Marital Status						
Married	3.5	28.6	47.3	20.6		
Not married	7.9	26.1	45.7	20.4	5.51	.138
Annual Household Income						
Less than $7,500	10.9	31.4	42.9	14.7		
$7,500–9,999	5.5	30.3	44.0	20.2		
$10,000–14,999	3.0	30.8	47.4	18.8		
$15,000 or more	0.0	15.8	38.3	45.9	39.35	.000
Education						
8 years or less	7.0	37.3	42.7	13.0		
9–11 years	7.6	26.8	46.8	19.0		
12 years	2.9	23.7	48.2	25.2		
13 years or more	3.5	16.5	51.3	28.7	28.75	.000
Home Ownership						
Own	4.0	28.4	47.1	20.6		
Rent	11.8	23.5	44.5	20.2	11.32	.015
Length of Residence in Community						
1–25 years	2.2	27.8	34.4	35.6		
26–50 years	3.5	29.4	49.8	17.4		
51–70 years	7.7	27.0	48.5	16.8		
71 or more years	8.2	23.6	48.2	20.0	22.86	.006
Service Knowledge						
None	10.7	32.1	39.3	17.9		
1 or 2	7.0	35.1	44.7	13.2		
3 or 4	6.0	27.2	47.2	19.6		
5 or more	3.4	22.4	48.3	25.9	14.75	.100

[a] All data in percents.

non-metropolitan rural and urban elders are less likely to be classified as "care dependent" than the metropolitan suburban or central city elderly residents. Yet, whereas 84 percent of the nonmetropolitan urban elderly population are completely independent only 72 percent of the nonmetropolitan rural elderly are so classified. This finding underscores the inadequacy and possible inaccuracy of using only a two-fold rural versus urban classification scheme and of operationalizing "rural" as all those places located outside metropolitan areas—i.e., nonmetropolitan. Clearly, there is considerable diversity within non-metropolitan and metropolitan populations that has not been sufficiently captured in much of the existing research.

In addition, as also was suggested earlier, multivariate analysis did reveal a different picture regarding rural versus urban elderly health dependence than was found with simple crosstabulations. When characteristics of elderly persons are entered into a regression analysis along with their community of residence, community type is no longer a significant predictor of health dependence, at least for the sample studied here. The apparent rural advantage in health dependency is most likely due to the greater percentages of whites, married, and elders who live with others in the sample. This finding suggests that previous studies purporting to uncover rural versus urban health differences have not necessarily demonstrated that community size or type has an independent effect on health. And this is a central question. Does living in places of lesser or greater rurality significantly affect the health experiences of elderly people who are otherwise similar in terms of sociodemographic characteristics?

One of the major areas that is often seen as differentiating rural versus urban areas and should be considered here is that of health services. There seems to be little disagreement in the literature that rural areas have fewer health resources and services and a lower ratio of doctors, nurses, pharmacists, and other health care personnel than do urban areas [15, 22]. Not only are health care services less available in rural areas, those that exist are less accessible [22]. Recall that many of the items in the health dependency index used in this research refer to the use of health care services. Thus, the lower health dependency scores found for the rural elderly respondents in this study may reflect a rural health service availability and accessibility disadvantage and not better health. In other words, the rural elderly population may have worse health but the dependent variable adopted in this study is more a measure of health service use which is lower.

However, this hypothesis cannot be directly tested with the data at hand, and an examination of the role played by health service availability and accessibility in rural versus urban elderly health dependency is further complicated by difficulties in establishing the direction of causal relationships in health related factors and by the fact that people may use health services outside their community of residence. But these observations do raise significant research questions in need of further investigation.

But it should also be noted that the data reveal an absence of community type differences in the self-assessed health of the sample studied here. This finding can be seen as independent confirmation of the position that health dependence is not simply an artifact of service availability and accessibility. However, some authors have suggested that a lack of rural versus urban elderly differences on subjective indicators of health, income, and housing adequacy may exist despite objective or "real" rural differences [23]. Thus, while the findings reported here do not support a thesis of rural elderly health dependency disadvantage, it would be ill-advised to conclude that this thesis can be rejected. Several concerns in regard to the data analyzed in this study have been identified. In addition, the sample used in this research comes from a rather small geographic area and the study is cross-sectional. No data was collected on length of health dependency or changes in same over time.

Finally, it must be remembered that the question of rural versus urban elderly health dependence differences is only a small part of the larger issue of health status and the response to health problems. Researchers should proceed in their investigation of community variations in health status and dependency, and, it is hoped, future work will benefit by a consideration of some of the points raised in this chapter. But questions about the outcomes and cost of health services for the elderly people in rural versus urban areas should also be clarified and pursued. These responses to health problems and the myriad of social, economic, biological, and attitudinal factors that interact to shape the health status of the elderly population must be more thoroughly examined in the rural versus urban context and for rural versus rural variations as well. Failing this, gerontologists will not move beyond a relatively descriptive level regarding the impact of community of residence on health and health-related behavior.

REFERENCES

1. G. Nelson, Social Services to the Urban and Rural Aged: The Experience of Area Agencies on Aging, *The Gerontologist, 20,* pp. 200-207, 1980.
2. E. G. Youmans and D. Larson, *Problems of Rural Elderly Households in Powell County, Kentucky,* Economic, Statistics, and Cooperative Services, United States Department of Agriculture, Washington, D.C., 1977.
3. E. G. Youmans, Health Orientations of Older Rural and Urban Men, *Geriatircs,* pp. 139-147, 1967.
4. A. J. Auerbach, The Elderly in Rural Areas: Differences in Urban Areas and Implications for Practice, in *Social Work in Rural Communities: A Book of Readings,* H. H. Ginsberg (ed.), Council on Social Work Education, New York, 1976.
5. Ecosometrics, *Review of Reported Differences between the Rural and Urban Elderly: Status, Needs, Services, and Service Costs,* Final report to the Administration on Aging, Washington, D.C., 1981.
6. E. G. Youmans, Age Group, Health, and Attitudes, *The Gerontologist, 14,* pp. 249-254, 1974.

7. V. R. Kivett and J. P. Scott, *The Rural By-Passed Elderly: Perspectives on Status and Needs,* Technical Bulletin No. 260, North Carolina Agricultural Research Service, Greensboro, North Carolina, 1979.
8. L. Paringer, J. Black, J. Feder, and J. Holahan, *Health Status and Use of Medical Services: Evidence on the Poor, Black, and Rural Elderly,* The Urban Institute, Washington, D.C., 1979.
9. K. Schooler, A Comparison of Rural and Non-Rural Elderly on Selected Variables, in *Rural Environments and Aging,* R. Atchley and T. O. Byerts (eds.), The Gerontological Society, Washington, D.C., 1975.
10. J. McCoy and D. Brown, Health Status among Low-Income Elderly Persons: Rural/Urban Differences, *Social Security Bulletin, 41,* pp. 14-26, 1978.
11. J. Dahlstein and J. C. Shank, Chronic and Acute Disease Problems in Rural Nursing Home Patients, *Journal of the American Geriatrics Society, 33,* pp. 681-687, 1979.
12. B. L. Ellenbogen, Health Status of the Rural Aged, in *Older Rural Americans,* E. G. Youmans (ed.), University of Kentucky Press, Lexington, 1967.
13. E. Palmore, Health Care Needs of the Rural Elderly, *International Journal of Aging and Human Development, 18,* pp. 39-45, 1983.
14. J. E. Burkhardt, et al., *Techniques for Translating Units of Need into Units of Service: The Case of Transportation and Nutrition Services for the Elderly,* unpublished paper, Administration on Aging, Washington, D.C., 1977.
15. W. R. Lassey and M. L. Lassey, The Physical Health Status of the Rural Elderly, in *The Elderly in Rural Society,* R. Coward and G. Lee (eds.), Springer, New York, 1985.
16. R. Ward, *The Aged Experience,* Harper and Row, New York, 1984.
17. B. Soldo, America's Elderly in the 1980s, *Population Bulletin, 35,* pp. 15-18, 1980.
18. L. Branch, Vulnerable Elders, Gerontological Society of America, Washington, D.C., 1980.
19. R. Andersen, J. Kravitz, and O. W. Anderson, *Equity in Health Services,* Ballinger, Cambridge, 1975.
20. R. Andersen, J. Lion, and O. W. Anderson, *Two Decades of Health Services: Social Survey Trends in Use Expenditure,* Ballinger, Cambridge, 1976.
21. J. A. Krout, Utilization of Services by the Elderly, *Social Service Review, 58,* pp. 281-290, 1984.
22. J. A. Krout, *The Aged in Rural America,* Greenwood Press, Wesport, Connecticut, 1986.
23. G. R. Lee and M. L. Lassey, Rural-Urban Differences among the Elderly: Economic, Social, and Subjective Factors, *Journal of Social Issues, 36,* pp. 62-74, 1980.

Chapter 8

SOCIAL DIMENSIONS OF MENTAL ILLNESS AMONG RURAL ELDERLY POPULATIONS

Jon Hendricks
and
Howard B. Turner

MENTAL HEALTH AMONG THE RURAL ELDERLY:
THE ISSUES

As popular wisdom has it, elderly people and elderly people who live in rural areas in particular, are at increased risk for mental illness. Both support and refutation for this view can be found in abundance [1, 2]. One key finding to emerge from the literature is a link between physical and mental illness. There is considerable evidence to suggest that rural aged persons experience symptoms of physical ill-health at a rate significantly higher than is typically the case among their age peers in general. The obvious question then, is, do they also show higher rates of emotional distress?

This chapter seeks to explore this mental health issue by examining four basic questions: Does the evidence indicate there is an increased incidence of mental illness among the elderly population as opposed to the general population? Is the rural elderly population at greater risk for mental illness than their urban counterparts? If not, what, if any, incidence patterns can be identified? Finally, what possible explanations might there be for the patterns which are encountered, and what research questions do they suggest?

Since definitions of mental illness and mental health are much debated, we begin by examining the underlying dimensions of these disputes and their implications for a discussion of the mental health of rural elderly persons. We next review the existing literature on incidence patterns of mental illness, and pose the causal questions raised. The subsequent three sections focus on the lifeworld of rural elderly people and its potential implications for mental health. We then briefly summarize some original empirical research on depression in a predominately rural state, and conclude by drawing out the implications of our findings for future research.

WHAT IS MENTAL HEALTH?

Perspectives on Mental Status

In discussing diverse perspectives on mental health, Mechanic identifies several distinct trends [3]. The "disease model" parallels the physician's conception of physical illness. Mental illness is a disease entity *sui generis* and treated as an endogenous condition stemming from neurophysiological or neurochemical causes. Alternately, a "developmental model" explains mental illness in terms of previous experiences leading to an existing problem. The presence of mental illness is thus seen as an outgrowth of experience. A "social reform model" assumes personality to be completely malleable; therefore, to correct a personality disorder, social injustices and inequities must be ameliorated. Finally, Mechanic outlines a "social conceptions" model in which illness is recognized within a particular milieu so that evaluations must only be made within the parameters established by that context.

Implicit in Mechanic's fourfold typology are a number of major disputes regarding the status of mental illness. Rather than dwelling on the intricacies of each of these in turn, we will briefly survey the lines along which they are drawn (see Figure 1). To begin with, we have the debate between what has been variously called the "medical," "biomedical," or "disease" model and more social-psychologically derived perspectives. Within the latter there is considerable discussion as to whether mental status is objective or whether it is socially constructed. Among those who see mental status as real, some contend it arises from psychologically-based phenomena, others from social factors, and yet others from interaction between the two. Among those who view mental status as socially constructed there are also a variety of interpretations. For some mental illness is a myth: what are essentially only normal variations of behavior or minor abnormalities are highlighted and labeled as indications of mental illness, snaring the stigmatized person in a web of social response which impels him/her into a career as a mental patient [4-7]. An alternative position, "social response theory" adopts an intermediate position [4]. Psychiatric dysfunction is real enough, but social responses magnify and perpetuate the dysfunction [4, 8]. Cultural relativism, closely aligned with Mechanic's "social conceptions" model, views mental illness as having meaning only within subcultures.

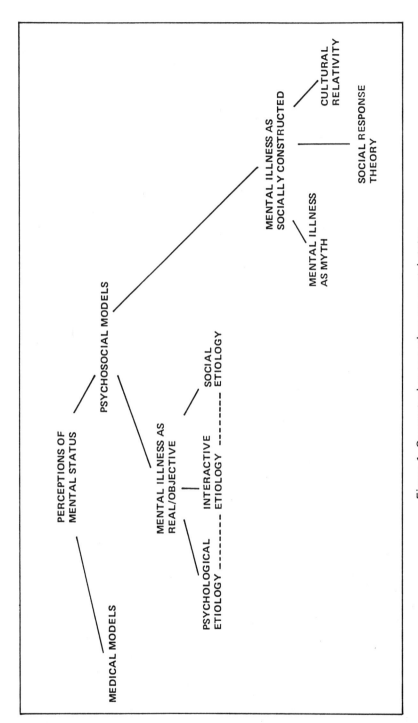

Figure 1. Conceptual perspectives on mental status

In the history of these disputes, these models have often been cast as opposing paradigms, each seen in opposition to the others. There has been a growing realization in some quarters, however, that in many respects they may not be contradictory, but complementary, and should be synthesized. Lazare for one, has endeavored to show how medical, psychological, behavioral, and social models of illness may actually complement one another in clinical practice [9]. Fabrega's ethnomedical approach also focuses on ways illness is socially constructed, interpreted, and handled, whether it is rooted in the physiological or not [10, 11]. Similarly, a unified systems perspective is dialectical, viewing illness as a process, in which physiological, psychological, cultural, and social levels interact [12, 13]. As early as 1942, Ackerknecht, in his cross-cultural work, developed a practical relative framework. He distinguished between autonormal and autopathological— what is seen as normal or pathological within a particular culture or subculture- and heteronormal or heteropathological—what is seen as normal or abnormal by outsiders [14]. An illustration of the first can be seen in the definitions of mental status by older or rural people themselves. The latter is illustrated by interpretations of the same phenomena by, say, psychiatrists brought in to evaluate older rural people. As we will see below, such a multidimensional approach and its causal framework may be usefully borne in mind in analyzing mental health issues among the rural elderly population.

For the remainder of this chapter and for purposes of discussion, we have chosen to focus on depression, since it is a condition in which the levels intertwine. Despite the diagnostic distinction between endogenous and reactive depressions presented in the DSM-III, in real life the demarcation is not all that clear. It seems apparent that mental status is a dialectical process, involving a multitude of levels. It is clear that some forms of mental dysfunction are primarily determined by one particular level, although they still interact with others. Organic brain syndromes are a case in point: they are obviously rooted the physiological, yet they are given meaning at a thoroughly social level. Or, alternately, certain forms of neurosis are more clearly functional in nature but may entail altered bodily processes.

INCIDENCE OF DEPRESSION AMONG ELDERLY PEOPLE

Gerontological research addressing possible relationships between age and mental health is inconsistent [15]. On the one hand, there is a sizeable literature maintaining that no identifiable relationship exists. In their landmark review to 1969, Dohrenwend and Dohrenwend assert that no significant tie between age and psychological disorder had been demonstrated [16]. Numerous empirical studies concur. Neither Tessler and Mechanic [17], nor Blazer and Williams [18] discovered any age-based connection in their search for causes of psychological distress among widely disparate samples. In a study of rural Canadians, Beiser also failed to uncover any reliable association between age and the affect scales he utilized [19]. Similarly, Andrews et al. concluded psychiatric illness was independent of age among their sample of Australians [20]. Conversely, a number of equally credible studies maintain that there is a relationship and that peak rates for significant symptoms of mental illness range between 15 and 25 percent among those over age sixty-five [2, 21-23].

As difficult as it is to reach consensus concerning the extent of mental illness among the general elderly population, it is even more difficult to find useful data dealing with those who live in rural areas. Despite the burgeoning literature that has grown up in the ten years since Youmans indicated that relatively little was known about rural old people [24], little attention has focused on the mental health of this group and the ways it may correlate with physical health and environmental or other risk factors. One might hypothesize, however, that the rates of mental illness will be no lower than for the aged population in general. In fact, given the overall harsher quality of life experienced by rural elderly persons when compared to their urban counterparts, the higher rate of impaired physical functioning and the mounting evidence questioning the overall patterns of better perceived mental health in rural areas [25], it would not be surprising to find the rate of mental disorder significantly higher.

When the focus is narrowed to look specifically at the prevalence of depression among the elderly people, the statistics become somewhat more informative. The literature in general suggests that, following a long plateau across the majority of adult life, the incidence of depression does increase incrementally in the later years, but probably not significantly until the decade of the seventies. Contrary to popular opinion, there is little evidence to indicate an acute midlife crisis, empty nest neuroses, or any trauma resulting from retirement that causes depression to come automatically tumbling after. Depression may result from losses, to be sure [26], and the losses of later life are no less poignant than any other. Yet epidemiologists remind us that the largest majority of elderly people—from 50 to 80 percent—do not experience any psychiatric impairment [15, 27, 28]. In other words, older persons are at most only at slightly greater risk for depression than is the population as a whole. At the same time, depressive reactions are the most frequent type of mental illness found among elderly people, with up to 4 percent of males and 11 percent of females over the age of sixty manifesting what could be described as moderate to severe symptoms [15, 23]. Based on a large-scale survey, Murrell, Himmelfarb and Wright found that rates increased significantly for males after age fifty-five, reaching approximately 14 percent [2]. Among similar aged females the relationship was curvilinear but climbed rapidly during and after middle age until 18 percent of the females showed some form of depression. Another comprehensive community-based study reports that although nearly 15 percent of those sixty-five or older showed substantial depressive symptoms, only 2 percent showed symptoms of primary depressive disorders [18].

While some investigators have recently argued that the rate of depression among elderly people may be estimated at too high a level due to misinterpretation of somatic complaints common to the aging process [28, 29], there is a countervailing opinion that these figures are too low, due to confounding with physical complaints and conditions. In fact, Gurland implies that psychiatrists have a bias resulting in underdiagnosis of late life depression [30]. According to Gurland, psychiatrists are more alert to symptoms of depression in younger groups, and are somewhat myoptic in their view of age; because of this, and because elderly people are commonly reluctant to admit depression, Gurland feels these symptoms may be dismissed as somatic complaints or concomitants of the normal aging process. Epstein makes a similar point when he asserts that depression in the people may be seen as a form of dementia, overlooked because of the masking of concurrent physical symptoms, or deemed just another facet of aging [31].

Detailed information on depression among rural populations is virtually unavailable, however [2]. Some researchers have even referred to attempts to assess real rural prevalence rates as an exercise in futility because field studies often suffer from conceptual as well as methodological difficulties [2]. More often than not, they focus on either a rural-urban dichotomy or adult age differences in mental well-being but not on a cross-classification of rates. As recently as the beginning of the 1980s, Hirschfeld and Cross were unable to locate any significant reports of depressive syndromes among the rural aged population or any urban-rural comparisons [32]. They did, however, find a few studies dealing with the question of depressive symptoms, though the data are limited. Recent empirical work comparing urban and non-urban differences in rates of depression for men and women found that there were no differences in rates of depression between rural and urban women, while significantly higher rates were observed among older men living in non-urban settings [2]. Although this sample was comprised of over 2500 persons, all those over age fifty-five were lumped together, thus including a decade of persons not normally defined as elderly by the gerontological literature.

Despite the difficulties of distinguishing between reactive versus endogenous states, there can be little doubt that depression among elderly people is reflective of their physical health, social situation, and other risk factors. It is a complicated relationship, to be sure, and it is an unwarranted assumption that the incidence of depression increases as a direct consequence of age. Indeed, among older people who are healthy and socially advantaged, depression may be no more common than among any other segment of the population. Rather, the notable increase may come among those chafing under the imposition of chronic ill health or among those attempting to cope with late life deprivations [2, 15, 18].

The Web of Causation

Physical illness is said by many to be the strongest source of distress and dissatisfaction among people in any age group [28, 33]. Despite a wide disparity in the measures utilized and in the strength of the relationship between physical health and mental health, its direction, or the specific nature of causal factors, there is emerging consensus that health and psychological well-being are intimately related. In a review of eighty-one empirical studies testing for a relationship between physical status and subjective well-being, Zautra and Hempel found that while slightly greater weight should be assigned to perceived as opposed to actual health, the two are correlated in a direct and consistent fashion with mental status, even after controlling for indirect and spurious associations [34]. As to what the underlying basis of this association might be, they are cautious and reticent, suggesting only a conditional relationship moderated by a variety of personal resources. Interestingly, they do acknowledge the relationship may run counter to the direction usually assumed: that a sense of well-being and satisfaction is predictive of physical health. Lawton reiterates the same point, highlighting three crucial questions which must be dealt with before any conclusions can be drawn: what is health; what is subjective well-being; and what are the mechanisms linking the two [35]?

Objective circumstances have also been identified as major factors in emotional distress. Perhaps the most consistent of these is the tie between lower socio-economic status and psychopathology in all its various forms [16, 32, 36, 37]. In their early overview, Dohrenwend and Dohrenwend pointed out consistency with which socio-economic variables are inversely related to psychological disorders [16]. In a similar vein, a number of investigators have gone a step further, specifying the types of psychological symptoms found among diverse status groupings [38-40]. A recent longitudinal investigation, this one a ten-year follow-up of survivors in a community survey, concluded that socio-economic factors are consistently strong predictors of various types of functioning, including mental health, among the old-old group [41]. There have been a number of attempts to ferret out just what part each SES component plays in psychological distress. Kessler found the relative importance of SES components to vary with sex and labor force status [42]. Yet each of the major components—income, education and occupational status—was significantly associated with distress, net of the other two. Husaini et al. found lack of education to be the most consistent predictor of psychiatric impairment [43]. Income, in and of itself, has also been found to be inversely related to impairment, but not as consistently. Occupational status per se, on the other hand, has not been found to be significantly linked to mental disorder [43]. In a one-year longitudinal study designed to evaluate changes in mental health status of elderly persons, education was used as a proxy for SES and was found to be one of two variables with greater than minimal predictive power [44].

Several recent studies have looked specifically at correlates of depression among the aging population. In their effort to unravel the causal patterns, Blazer and Williams found high rates of social and economic resource impairment among elderly clients to be predictive of both depressive symptoms and disorders [18].

Murrell, Himmelfarb and Wright concurred, though they noted that SES was more predictive for women over the age of fifty-five than for men [2]. The point is, when faced with a dearth of material resources, diagnosis of depressive conditions becomes more probable.

This issue has been the subject of lengthy and involved debates. Briefly, the major hypotheses regarding the inverse relationship between SES and mental disorder may be summarized as follows. Some contend that people of lower socio-economic status are more subject to deprivation and distress, resulting from such things as a lack of basic necessities and health resources, poor living conditions, economic worries, and the attenuation of autonomy and personal initiative [45-47]. Consequently, they manifest higher rates of psychological disorder. Others argue that there is a greater disposition to mental illness in persons of lower socio-economic status because impairment secondary to mental disorder causes a drift down the socio-economic scale. Furthermore, the level of predisposition may be maintained by associative mating [48]. A third approach asserts that people of lower SES form distinct subcultures with their own set of behavioral expectations. Due to intercultural differences, there is a greater tendency on the part of psychiatrists to label them as more severely mentally ill. Still others contend that when persons of lower SES have psychological problems, they are treated differently, both in terms of treatment received (or absence of it) and in the reactions of others. These responses tend to be pejorative, aggravating and perpetuating mental disorder [49].

IMPLICATIONS FOR THE RURAL ELDERLY

Each of the factors discussed above as exacerbating the risk for depression is known to vary by age. They have also been shown to differentiate among people in rural areas. To illustrate, Berry points out that adaptive success for either groups or for individuals is relative to their personal resources and external components of the rural setting [50]. Similarly, Lawton employs the notion of "environmental press" to explain individual adjustment and adaptation [51]. Those individuals possessed of greater resources promoting resiliency in the face of potentially disruptive situational variables demonstrate greater adaptation. In the view of Nahemow and Lawton, individuals with relatively high levels of personal competence can adapt to a wider range of environmental press possibilities, including stressors, thereby avoiding risk of behavioral or psychological disruption [52]. The most efficient and effective adaptation occurs when moderate levels of press are present relative to competence. On almost all objective criteria indicating access to those resources thought to promote life satisfaction, rural elderly people fare less well than their urban counterparts. Study after study of rural life have indicated an erosion of traditional sources of social support, quality of life, and factors relevant for life satisfaction among those who grow old in rural areas. To cite but one example, in summarizing a variety of statistics gathered by the

National Center for Health Statistics on physical health in rural populations, Palmore maintains that rural elderly people suffer one-fourth more acute health conditions, and have more chronic limitations, than the average older person [53]. The severity of the rural physical environments is thought to be both stressful and causally responsible [54-58].

The Life Situation of Rural Elderly People

To appreciate the full range of factors affecting the mental status of the rural elderly people, it is essential to have some grasp of the living conditions they face. Rural life, despite its stereotypic peacefulness, pastoral calm, and independent lifestyle, can be beset with considerable harshness. Age and locale potentially impose a double jeopardy on rural elderly persons [59]. The economic realities of rurality reveal inequities of the first order. Despite efforts over the years to improve the economic well-being of the nation's rural population, they continue to lag behind their urban counterparts in terms of average income and percentage living in or near poverty [60, 61]. The number of rural persons living at, or below, the poverty level increased from 9.9 million in 1979 to 13.5 million in 1983, a 36 percent increase in four years [62]. The non-urban poverty rate of older persons is some 70 percent higher than among these living in cities [63, 64]. Lower educational levels and higher drop-out rates are also characteristic of rural persons.

Housing is another problematic area. Although they are more likely to own their own homes, residences of rural elderly people are less well-equipped, in a worse state of repair, and more likely to have structural and/or electrical deficiencies [60, 65]. A greater percentage lack adequate plumbing, complete kitchens, adequate drinking water supplies and satisfactory sewage systems than in nearly any urban area of the country [66, 67]. Of the 3 million substandard dwellings in the country occupied by older persons, 40 percent are clustered in metropolitan or rural areas [68]. The situation has not improved as we move into the latter years of the 1980s; if anything, rural elderly people now live in even more debilitated circumstances [69].

The provision of health care adds yet another prejudicial dimension to the life circumstances of rural persons. To begin with, estimates indicate that physician case loads are two to five times higher in rural areas. Even when community health-care facilities are available, they are qualitatively less adequate than in urban areas [70]. On almost every dimension, rural health care is less advantageous than in urban areas; the availability of specialists, especially mental health specialists, is not weighted toward the rural population.

Health care is also severely restricted in that even when services are available, distance and transportation difficulties hinder access to acceptable health care [71]. Transportation problems are compounded for rural elderly persons because public transport is virtually nonexistent [72]. As a consequence, the number of physician visits is below that found in urban areas, even though the incidence of chronic conditions, their multiplicity, and restrictions resulting from these conditions is higher. Further, many of the social services supportive of urban elderly persons are largely absent on the rural scene. Like health services, critics maintain that even those social services which are present are of lower quality [73].

Life Satisfaction of Rural Elderly People

Provided there is a relationship between living conditions and life satisfaction among both urban and rural elderly people, the inequities described above should predict lower levels of subjective well-being and a higher incidence of psychological distress. Research on urban populations has revealed exactly that: the more dire the living conditions, the less favorable is life satisfaction in general and mental status in particular [74]. There is a curious irony, however, in the way older rural persons perceive themselves and their situation. Study after study has shown that rural elderly people are at least as satisfied with their lives as their urban counterparts. In a compilation of research through the 1970s, Larson noted few if any differences in aggregate life-satisfaction levels found in urban and rural older populations in spite of the less favorable objective conditions of the latter [75]. Other investigators take an even stronger stance, pointing to greater expressions of subjective well-being among rural elderly people despite the objective conditions and service deficiencies [76-79]. In an innovative project based on a compilation of four diverse data sets indexing the "degree of urbanism" via population size, Liang and Worfel showed urbanism to be a polytomous variable having both indirect and interactive effects on their elderly sample's life satisfaction through health and objective and subjective social integration [80]. In their discussion of their results, Liang and Worfel contend that concepts of urbanism should be multidimensional, focusing on environmental characteristics as well as crucial dimensions of subjective perceptions and social relationships.

Finally, the stability of values represents another dimension of the question of mental status. In light of what some regard as the greater displacement of traditional values in rural areas resulting from the impact of modernization and the influx of mass communications, it is indeed surprising that mental health has not declined. Broadly speaking, rural values are "traditional," characterized as involving a complex of themes: fatalism; and orientation to concrete places and things; personal and kinship relations as a source of well-being; and an emphasis on *being* rather than *doing* [25]. Larson describes a similar set of values for both groups, yet he maintains that though urban and rural values are changing in a similar direction, the magnitude and the rate of change is such that differentials between the two are actually increasing [75]. Ansello echoes a similar view by asserting that a strong sense of community competence, suspiciousness of government, and a fatalistic view of history are central attitudes for rural elderly people [81]. As a consequence, they may have a stronger desire to contribute rather than receive support or assistance from interpersonal ties; this perhaps accounts at least in part for their underutilization of services even when they are available [82].

DATA ON RURAL MENTAL HEALTH

These, then, are the factors which must be taken into account in any discussion of rural mental health. Despite conditions which among urban populations would be predicative of emotional difficulties, rural elderly people apparently do not fare too poorly. Objective disadvantages aside, levels of life satisfaction and subjective well-being of rural elderly persons suggest that they have resources which help insulate them from the spectre of depression or other manifestations of mental illness.

Sample and Method

To help illuminate any possible connections between rurality and depression, we collected empirical data in a statewide survey in a predominantly rural state. In late 1984, 1078 persons aged eighteen and over were selected by random digit dialing and queried in a telephone survey administered as part of a periodic poll conducted by the University of Kentucky Survey Research Center. Every phone in the state had an equal opportunity of being called. Overall our response rate was 68.9 percent, yielding a sample of 743. The potential sampling error is + or 3.7 percent at a 95 percent confidence interval. Our analyses suggest the sample is generally representative of the population of the state and is not significantly biased. The percentage of respondents over the age of sixty-five ($N = 118$) is virtually identical to the state average at 10.4. On such variables as sex, education, and income, the sample appears representative; only on race is our non-white distribution of approximately 6 percent less than that of the state as a whole. Nonetheless, we are confident that our data are acceptable in customary survey terms.

Data for this portion of our analyses are derived from an abbreviated version of the eighteen-item Center for Epidemiological Studies Depression Scale (CES-D). Since its development, the assessment instrument has been widely used on a variety of age groups in telephone and personal interviews, and has been found to be a reliable instrument [83]. Six items,[1] previously noted to have the highest correlations with the total scale [2] were selected. In our investigation all six items were found via a factor analysis, to load heavily on a single factor, thus indicating unidimensionality. In our research the six items were tested for the highest item-scale correlation and found to have an alpha reliability of 0.85. Further, our

---

[1] The six items were: "shake the blues;" "felt depressed;" "been happy;" "felt lonely;" "enjoy life;" "felt sad"—response codes adjusted for scale construction. Alpha = .85372.

results indicate that the abbreviated scale effectively discriminated across various subgroups of the population.

In addition to the CES-D scale, we ascertained physical health by means of the Physical Health Index (PMI) developed by Berkman and Breslow [84]. This tool combines thirty-seven items dealing with levels of energy, symptoms, chronic conditions, impairments, and disabilities into an overall measure of health scored from high energy levels with no complaints (1) to severe disability (7). Independent assessments of reliability and congruence with physician ratings have been reported to be more than acceptable [85, 86]. Demographic data collected include sex, education, family, race, income, age, and educational levels. Place of residence was established both in terms of self-perceived rurality and actual county, this latter enable us to verify rural residence.

Results

Although there is not room here to present a detailed description of all our findings, we can summarize by noting that bivariate correlation coefficients suggest there is virtually no shared variation between depression and age or between depression and place of residence. When the scale items were dichotomized to indicate "at risk" and "not at risk" for depression, a cross tabular analysis indicated that neither place of residence (rural vs. non-rural), age, nor sex were statistically associated with likelihood of depression. Application of a *t*-test to ascertain any possible relationship between race and global assessments of mental health as measured by the abbreviated CES-D scale also proved to be non-significant. Nonwhites did show marginally higher mean scores, suggestive of a greater incidence of depression; however, because of our small number of non-white respondents they were deleted from further analysis.

In an attempt to determine which factors might be suppressing possible relationships, a series of first-order partial correlations were run. The findings (see Table 1) suggest that income, education, sex, and health all exert varying degrees of influence upon the correlations of interest. All correlations were in the direction anticipated and from moderately to highly significant. The strongest suppressor, by far, is health. With an *r* of 12.6 = -.15 the connection is significant at the .001 level. This is further confirmed by fourth-order correlations including all control variables. Interestingly, we found that when health is held constant, there is actually an inverse relationship between age and depression. It is particularly important, we believe, to note the influence of sex on this unexpected age-depression correlation when health is controlled. Although both males and females contributed to the inverse relationships, the male correlation (-.06) was not statistically significant while the female correlation (-.18) was highly significant (.00). Although our data are not conclusive, this finding is certainly deserving of further attention by other investigators.

Table 1. Partial Correlations Between (1) CES-Depression
Scale and (2) Age, Controlling for (3) Sex, (4) Income,
(5) Education, and (6) Physical Health Index

r_{12}	=	-0.00
$r_{12.3}$	=	-0.06^{*}
$r_{12.4}$	=	-0.08^{**}
$r_{12.5}$	=	-0.08^{**}
$r_{12.6}$	=	-0.15^{***}
$r_{12.3456}$	=	-0.19^{***}

$^{*} p < .05$
$^{**} p < .01$
$^{***} p < .001$

To assess the relative influence of the five individual variables shown in the table upon depression, net of the others, we also ran a multiple regression analysis. The results are presented in Table 2 and, as can be seen, health again shows up as having a strong influence on depressive symptoms. Once more, with the influence of health controlled, age is shown to be significantly stronger but negatively related to depression, as are income and sex (females higher). Interestingly, education was discovered to have relatively little influence when the other factors were controlled. In no instance were we able to discriminate between rural and urban locales of our respondents. The sole exception was when health remained uncontrolled: in this instance, rural residence did at first appear to be associated with higher depression scores. Initially this might be interpreted to imply that rural residents are indeed more prone to expressing depressive symptomatology, yet when health conditions were held constant, the relationship disappeared. At most these data can be said to suggest that no simple correlation exists between age and increased levels of depression or between rurality and mental status. What is apparent is that when physical health is impaired, as among elderly or rural residents, there does seem to be a somewhat higher risk of depression. This implication is consistent with the widespread pattern pointed to by Tessler and Mechanic in their secondary analyses of four diverse data sets [17]. It is also a point made by Aneshensel and her colleagues in their survey analysis of the reciprocal interaction between physical illness and depression [87].

In a state where the quality of life of elderly rural persons would suggest that by most so-called objective standards they are even more hard-pressed than are rural persons in general, the lack of a statistically significant relationship between place of residence and depression is perplexing. Obviously, there are factors operating that large-scale surveys of this type do not tap. Investigations of the impact of rurality upon mental health which do not control for the relevance of physical health indicators may well mistakenly suggest that those who live on farms or in small towns are at a greater risk. Clearly, closer specification of the relationship between at least these three factors is necessary before drawing conclusions.

Table 2. CES-Depression Scale Regressed on Physical Health Index,
Age, Income, Sex, and Education

Independent Variable	Unstandardized Coefficient	Standardized Coefficient	t-Value
Health	0.64	0.26	6.36**
Age	−0.05	−0.20	−4.76**
Income	−0.25	−0.15	−3.37**
Sex	−0.86	−0.12	−2.98*
Education	−0.16	−0.06	−1.36
(Intercept)	4.88		5.60**
r^2 (Adjusted)	0.12		
Standard Error	3.50		
N	621		

*$p < .01$
**$p < .001$

IMPLICATIONS AND SUGGESTIONS
FOR FUTURE RESEARCH

In attempting to explain the strong ties between physical and mental health, four alternative hypotheses come to mind. First, physical illness may stand as a direct causal antecedent of mental illness. Susceptibility notwithstanding, physical ill-health may trigger psychological and emotional disruptions. Certainly there is a large body of literature pointing to the impact of morbidity on mental status [88]. Second, the converse may also be the case: mental impairments translate into somatization and a greater susceptibility to physical illness. Allowing for a lag period of roughly four months, Aneshensel, Frerichs and Huba were able to identify what they construed as a causal link between mental to physical illness [87]. Third, the two may interact: impairments in either realm have a dialectical relationship with problems in the other. Alternatively, both physical and mental illness may be due to some other confounding or external factors. Among the antecedent causes shown to be implicated by previous research are SES, age, sex, and other demographic variables.

Then again, there is another possibility. Rather than looking at unifactorial explanations, we should redirect our attention to a multidimensional framework. Those factors Lawton and others lump under the general rubric of "environmental press" comprise a complex interweaving of physical, psychological, and socio-economic factors [51]. Illness, whether physical or mental, is a consequence of changes in systematic functioning, triggered by stressors which affect people differently, and which may be interpreted and responded to in various ways.

If this is indeed the case, the inverse relationship between age and depression pointed to by our data, and noted by other researchers as well, might be accounted for by the better coping mechanisms and strategies utilized by older persons. Or perhaps the lower incidence of mental illness and absence of physical impairments characteristic of the elderly people in our sample might stem from what could be described as the relative equanimity of life in the second half of adulthood; it might be that with age, people are less likely to feel stress or be buffeted by transitions which, at an earlier point in their lives, might have been more stressful. In other words, over the years people may develop coping strategies they did not possess earlier in life.

Obviously, how mental illness is conceptualized and what types of conditions are being looked for will influence the types of diagnoses made. What is appropriate in the context of urban lifestyles may verge on the irrelevant in rural situations. The same applies for the whole range of objective conditions thought to bring dire consequences for those who must adapt to them. Ackerknecht's contention regarding the distinction between autopathology and heteropathology is particularly germane for the rural elderly population [14]. Having grown old in the face of challenging physical environments, with conditions which might be regarded as inhospitable in metropolitan areas, older people simply do not evaluate themselves on their own mental status as an outsider would.

Unfortunately, one of the risks in making generalizations about urban and rural populations is that we may lose sight of the diversities. This danger seems particularly poignant when discussing rural residents and the issues with which they must cope. Almost by definition, or be default, rurality is treated as a homogeneous category. Clearly this is an inaccurate view. Willits and her colleagues point to the paucity of documentation of differences within rural life [89]. Such personal characteristics as age, race, ethnicity, income, and education are rarely considered to vary much at all. Even when discussing a single occupational category found in rural areas—farming, for example—considerable latitude is subsumed. Ignoring the cultural and environmental diversities among portions of America's elderly population can only jeopardize our ability to understand the patterning of their behavior.

If social scientists or service providers are to make a contribution in terms of understanding or intervention, they need to assume what the anthropological jargon refers to as an *emic* approach—an attempt to understand the situation of rural elderly people as they themselves experience and perceive it. The practical implications of such a suggestion range from the need for more qualitative studies utilizing careful conceptualizations of mental illness as seen by non-urban people themselves, to the development of appropriate interventions. We have commented on the under-utilization of health services, including mental health services in rural areas: Coward and Smith refer to the existence of a "treatment gap" resulting from either physical or social-psychological barriers [90]. Part of the reason for such a gap may be that urban service models abrade the values and spirit of independence of rural dwellers. Even if actual programs are not transplanted, the conceptual models in the identification of depression and its causes which have been transported may miss the dynamic of the dialectical relationship characteristic of rural environments. Scheidt's admonition to become familiar with rural values, community structure, and perception of life events prior to offering service delivery, intervention models, or conceptualizations, applies particularly to all aspects of the assessment of mental status [91].

To note that rural mental illness prevalence rates are no higher than urban rates is not the same as saying that little or no psychological distress exists. It may be masked, it may be accepted and not verbalized, or it may not be labelled by the respondents themselves. Surely all locales can profit from better mental health services. While social policy changes designed to reshape the structure of services so as to enhance access to mental health care for rural elderly people are indicated, the rural elderly themselves should be involved in the creation of those programs. Rural service providers must learn to read between the lines, to see the world as their clients see it in order to offer optimum and effective assistance.

REFERENCES

1. B. S. Myers, B. Kalayam, and V. Mei-Tal, Late-onset Delusional Depression: A Distinct Clinical Entity, *Journal of Clinical Psychiatry, 45*, pp. 347-349, 1984.
2. S. A. Murrell, S. Himmelfarb, and K. Wright, Prevalence of Depression and Its Correlates in Older Adults, *American Journal of Epidemiology, 117*, pp. 173-185, 1983.
3. D. Mechanic, *Mental Health and Social Policy*, Prentice-Hall, New Jersey, 1980.
4. J. M. Murphy, Psychiatric Labeling in Cross-cultural Perspective, *Science, 191*, pp. 1019-1028, 1976.
5. T. Scheff, *Being Mentally Ill*, Aldine, Chicago, 1966.
6. T. Szasz, *The Myth of Mental Illness: Foundations of a Theory of Personal Conduct*, Hoeber-Harper Publishers, New York, 1969.
7. T. Szasz, The Myth of Mental Illness: Three Agenda, *Journal of Humanistic Psychology, 14*, pp. 11-19, 1974.
8. N. E. Waxler, Culture and Mental Illness: A Social Labeling Perspective, *Journal of Nervous and Mental Disease, 159*, pp. 379-395, 1974.
9. A. Lazare, Hidden Conceptual Models in Clinical Psychiatry, *New England Journal of Medicine, 288*, pp. 345-351, 1973.
10. H. Fabrega, The Scientific Usefulness of the Idea of Illness, *Perspectives in Biology and Medicine, 22*, pp. 554-558, 1979.
11. H. Fabrega, Culture and Psychiatric Illness: Biomedical and Ethnomedical Perspectives, in *Cultural Conceptions of Mental Health and Therapy*, A. J. Marsella and G. M. White (eds.), D. Reidel, Boston, 1984.
12. G. I. Engel, A Unified Concept of Health and Disease, *Perspectives in Biology and Medicine, 3*, pp. 459-485, 1960.

13. H. Fabrega, The Study of Disease in Relation to Culture, *Behavioral Science, 17*, pp. 183-203, 1972.

14. E. Ackerknecht, Psychopathology, Primitive Medicine and Primitive Culture, *Bulletin of the History of Medicine, 14*, pp. 30-69, 1942.

15. D. Blazer, The Epidemiology of Depression in Late Life, in *Depression and Aging*, L. D. Breslau and M. R. Haug (eds.), Springer Publishing, New York, 1983.

16. B. P. Dohrenwend and B. S. Dohrenwend, *Social Status and Psychological Disorder: A Causal Inquiry*, Wiley-Interscience, New York, 1969.

17. R. Tessler and D. Mechanic, Psychological Distress and Perceived Health Status, *Journal of Health and Social Behavior, 19*, pp. 254-262, 1978.

18. D. Blazer and C. D. Williams, Epidemiology of Dysphoria and Depression in an Elderly Population, *American Journal of Psychiatry, 137*, pp. 439-444, 1980.

19. M. Beiser, Components and Correlates of Mental Well-being, *Journal of Health and Social Behavior, 15*, pp. 320-327, 1974.

20. G. Andrews, et al., The Relation of Social Factors to Physical and Psychiatric Illness, *American Journal of Epidemiology, 108*, pp. 27-35, 1978.

21. G. M. Barrow and P. A. Smith, *Aging, The Individual, and Society* (2nd Edition), West Publishing Company, St. Paul, 1983.

22. Department of Health, Education and Welfare, The Federal Council on Aging, *Mental Health and the Elderly, Recommendations for Action*, U.S. Government Printing Office, Washington, D.C., 1979.

23. D. W. K. Kay and K. Bergman, Epidemiology of Mental Disorders Among the Aged in the Community, in *Handbook of Mental Health and Aging*, J. E. Birren and R. B. Sloane (eds.), Prentice-Hall, New Jersey, 1980.

24. E. G. Youmans, The Rural Aged, *The Annals of the American Academy of Political and Social Sciences, 429*, pp. 81-90, 1977.

25. National Institute of Mental Health, *Mental Health and Rural America: An Overview and Annotated Bibliography*, U.S. Government Printing Office, Washington, D.C., 1979.

26. R. N. Butler and M. I. Lewis, *Aging and Mental Health* (3rd Edition), C. V. Mosby Company, St. Louis, 1982.

27. L. K. George, D. G. Blazer, I. Winfield-Laird, P. J. Leaf, and R. Eischbach, Psychiatric Disorders and Mental Health Service Use in Later Life: Evidence from the Epidemiologic Catchment Area Program, in *Epidemiology in Late Life*, J . Brody and G. Maddox (eds.), Springer, New York, 1986.

28. A. Stoudemire and D. G. Blazer, Depression in the Elderly, in *Handbook of Depression*, E. E. Beckman and W. R. Leber (eds.), Dorsey Press, Homewood, Illinois, 1985.

29. J. M. Berry, M. Storandt, and A. Coyne, Age and Sex Differences in Somatic Complaints Associated with Depression, *Journal of Gerontology, 39*, pp. 465-467, 1984.

30. B. J. Gurland, The Comparative Frequency of Depression in Various Adult Age Groups, *Journal of Gerontology, 31*, pp. 283-292, 1976.

31. L. J. Epstein, Depression in the Elderly, Journal of Gerontology, 31, pp. 278-282, 1976.

32. R. M. A. Hirschfeld and C. K. Cross, Epidemiology of Affective Disorders: Psychosocial Risk Factors, *Archives of General Psychiatry, 39*, pp. 35-46, 1982.

33. J. Flanagan, A Research Approach to Improving Our Quality of Life, *American Psychologist, 33*, pp. 138-147, 1978.
34. A. Zautra and A. Hempel, Subjective Well-being and Physical Health: A Narrative Literature Review with Suggestions for Further Research, *International Journal of Aging and Human Development, 19*, pp. 95-110, 1984.
35. M. P. Lawton, Investigating Health and Subjective Well-being, *International Journal of Aging and Human Development, 19*, pp. 157-166, 1984.
36. M. Romaniuk, W. J. McAuley, and G. Arling, An Examination of the Prevalence of Mental Disorders Among the Elderly in the Community, *Journal of Abnormal Psychology, 92*, pp. 458-467, 1983.
37. B. P. Dohrenwend, Psychiatric Disorder in General Populations: Problem of the Untreated 'Case,' *American Journal of Public Health, 60*, pp. 1052-1064, 1970.
38. A. B. Hollingshead and F. C. Redlich, *Social Class and Mental Illness: A Community Study*, John Wiley and Sons, New York, 1958.
39. G. J. Warheit, C. E. Holzer III, and J. J. Schwab, An Analysis of Social Class and Racial Differences in Depressive Symptomatology: A Community Study, *Journal of Health and Social Behavior, 14*, pp. 291-299, 1973.
40. M. A. Liberman, Social Contexts of Depression, in *Depression and Aging*, L. D. Breslau and M. R. Haug (eds.), Springer Publishing Company, New York, 1983.
41. E. B. Palmore, J. B. Nowlin. and H. S. Wang, Predictors of Function Among the Old-Old: A 10-year Follow-up, *Journal of Gerontology, 40*, pp. 244-250, 1985.
42. R. C. Kessler, Socioeconomic Status and Psychological Distress, *American Sociological Review, 47*, pp. 752-764, 1982.
43. B. A. Husaini, J. A. Neff, and R. H. Stone, Psychiatric Impairment in Rural Communities, *Journal of Community Psychology, 7*, pp. 137-146, 1979.
44. M. Haug, L. Belgrave, and B. Gratton, Mental Health and the Elderly: Factors in Stability and Change Over Time, *Journal of Health and Social Behavior, 25*, pp. 110-115, 1984.
45. M. L. Kohn, The Interaction of Social Class and Other Factors in the Etiology of Schizophrenia, *American Journal of Psychiatry, 133*, pp. 177-180, 1976.
46. L. Srole, T. S. Langner, S. T. Michael, et al., *Mental Health in the Metropolis. The Midtown Manhattan Study*, McGraw-Hill, New York, 1962.
47. J. H. Abrahamson, et al., Indicators of Social Class: A Comparative Appraisal of Measures for Use in Epidemiological Studies, *Social Science and Medicine, 16*, pp. 1739-1746, 1982.
48. E. M. Godberg and S. L. Morrison, Schizophrenia and Social Class, *British Journal of Psychiatry, 109*, pp. 785-802, 1963.
49. J. J. Schwab and M. E. Schwab, *The Sociocultural Roots of Mental Illness: An Epidemiological Survey*, Plenum Press, New York, 1978.
50. J. W. Berry, Cultural Ecology and Individual Behavior, in *Human Behavior and Environment: Advances in Theory and Research, Vol. 4, Environment Culture*, I. Altman, A. Rapoport, and J. F. Wohlwill (eds.), Plenum Press, New York, 1980.
51. M. P. Lawton, The Impact of the Environment on Aging and Behavior, in *Handbook of the Psychology of Aging*, J. E. Birren and K. W. Schaie (eds.), Van Nostrand Reinhold, New York, 1977.

52. L. Nahemow and M. P. Lawton, Toward an Ecological Theory of Adaptation and Aging, in *Environmental Psychology. People and Their Physical Settings,* H. M. Proshansky, W. H. Ittelson, and L. G. Rivlin (eds.), Holt, Reinhart and Winston, New York, 1976.

53. E. B. Palmore, Health Care Needs of the Rural Elderly, *International Journal of Aging and Human Development, 18,* pp. 39-45, 1983-1984.

54. G. R. Lee and M. L. Lassey, The Elderly, in *Rural Society in the U.S.: Issues for the 1980s,* D. A. Dillman and D. J. Hobbs (eds.), Westview Press, Colorado, 1982.

55. R. T. Coward and G. R. Lee, An Introduction to Aging in Rural Environments, in *The Elderly in Rural Society,* R. T. Coward and G. R. Lee (eds.), Springer Publishing Company, New York, 1985.

56. P. G. Windley and R. J. Scheidt, The Well-being of Older Persons in Small Rural Towns: A Town Panel Approach, *Educational Gerontology, 5,* pp. 335-373, 1980.

57. P. G. Windley and R. J. Scheidt, An Ecological Model of Mental Health Among Small Town Rural Elderly, *Journal of Gerontology, 37,* pp. 235-242, 1982.

58. P. G. Windley and R. J. Scheidt, The Ecology of Aging, in *Handbook of the Psychology of Aging,* J. E. Birren and K. W. Schaie (eds.), Van Nostrand Reinhold, New York, 1985.

59. W. J. Goudy and C. Dobson, Work, Retirement and Financial Situation of the Rural Elderly, in *The Elderly in Rural Society,* R. T. Coward and G. R. Lee (eds.), Springer Publishing Company, New York, 1985.

60. D. A. Dillman and K. R. Tremblay, Jr., The Quality of Life in Rural America, *Annals, American Academy of Political and Social Sciences, 429,* pp. 115-130, 1977.

61. B. A. Chadwick and H. M. Bahr, Rural Poverty, in *Rural U.S.A. Persistence and Change,* T. R. Ford (ed.), Iowa State University Press, Ames, 1978.

62. J. Shotland, *Rising Poverty, Declining Health: Nutritional Status of the Rural Poor,* Public Voice for Food and Health Policy, Washington, D.C., 1986.

63. G. R. Lee and M. L. Lassey, Rural-Urban Differences Among the Elderly: Economic, Social and Subjective Factors, *Journal of Social Issues, 36,* pp. 62-74, 1980.

64. U.S. Census, *Statistical Abstract of the United States,* U.S. Government Printing Office, Washington, D.C., 1985.

65. E. W. Morris and M. Winter, Housing, in *Rural Society in the U.S.: Issues for the 1980s,* D. A. Dillman and D. J. Hobbs (eds.), Westview Press, Colorado, 1982.

66. R. J. Struyk, The Housing Situation of Elderly Americans, *The Gerontologist, 17,* pp. 130-139, 1977.

67. G. D. Arnold, *Housing of the Rural Elderly,* Economic Development Division, Economic Research Service, U.S. Department of Agriculture, Rural Development Research Report, 1984.

68. P. K. H. Kim, The Low Income Rural Elderly: Under-served Victims of Public Inequity, in *Toward Mental Health of the Rural Elderly,* P. K. H. Kim and C. P. Wilson (eds.), University Press of America, Washington, D.C., 1981.

69. R. A. Bylund, Rural Housing: Perspectives for the Aged, in *The Elderly in Rural Society,* R. F. Coward and G. R. Lee (eds.), Springer Publishing Company, New York, 1985.

70. K. D. Rainey and K. G. Rainey, Rural Government and Local Public Services, in *Rural U.S.A. Persistence and Change,* T. R. Ford (ed.), Iowa State University, Ames, 1978.

71. M. K. Miller, Health and Medical Care, in *Rural Society in the U.S.: Issues for the 1980s*, D. A. Dillman and D. J. Hobbs (eds.), Westview Press, Colorado, 1982.

72. W. R. Lassey and M. L. Lassey, The Physical Health Status of the Rural Elderly, in *The Elderly in Rural Society*, R. T. Coward and C. P. Lee (eds.), Springer Publishing Company, New York, 1985.

73. R. T. Coward and E. Rathbone-McCuan, Delivering Health and Human Services to the Elderly in Rural Society, in *The Elderly in Rural Society*, R. T. Coward and G. R. Lee (eds.), Springer Publishing Company, New York, 1985.

74. A. P. Fengler and L. Jensen, Perceived and Objective Conditions As Predictors of the Life Satisfaction of Urban and Nonurban Elderly, *Journal of Gerontology, 36*, pp. 750-752, 1981.

75. O. F. Larson, Values and Beliefs of Rural People, in *Rural U.S.A. Persistence and Change*, T. R. Ford (ed.), Iowa State University Press, Ames, 1978.

76. A. Campbell, P. E. Converse, and W. L. Rodgers, *The Quality of American Life: Perception, Evaluation, and Satisfaction*, Russel Sage Foundation, New York, 1976.

77. G. V. Donnenwerth, F. Guy, and M. J. Norvell, Life Satisfaction Among Older Persons: Rural-Urban and Racial Comparisons, *Social Science Quarterly, 59*, pp. 578-583, 1978.

78. J. M. Edward and D. L. Klemmack, Correlates of Life Satisfaction: A Reexamination, *Journal of Gerontology, 28*, pp. 497-502, 1973.

79. L. M. Hynson, Rural-Urban Differences in Satisfaction among the Elderly, *Rural Sociology, 40*, pp. 64-66, 1975.

80. J. Liang and B. L. Worfel, Urbanism and Life Satisfaction among the Aged, *Journal of Gerontology, 38*, pp. 97-106, 1983.

81. E. F. Ansello, Antecedent Principles in Rural Gerontology Education, in *Toward Mental Health of the Rural Elderly*, P. K. H. Kim and C. P. Wilson (eds.), University Press of America, Washington, D.C., 1981.

82. P. Shephard, *Rural Aged*, paper presented at the annual meeting of the Gerontological Society of America, San Antonio, Texas, November 1984.

83. C. S. Aneshensel, et al., Measuring Depression in the Community: A Comparison of Telephone and Personal Interviews, *Public Opinion Quarterly, 46*, pp. 119-126, 1982.

84. L. F. Berkman and L. Breslow, *Health and Ways of Living*, Oxford University Press, New York, 1983.

85. K. F. Ferraro, Self-ratings of Health among the Old and the Old-old, *Journal of Health and Social Behavior, 21*, pp. 377-383, 1980.

86. G. G. Fillenbaum, Social Context and Self-assessments of Health Among the Elderly, *Journal of Health and Social Behavior, 20*, pp. 45-51, 1979.

87. C. S. Aneshensel, R. R. Frerichs, and G. J. Huba, Depression and Physical Illness: A Multiwave, Nonrecursive Causal Model, *Journal of Health and Social Behavior, 25*, pp. 350-371, 1984.

88. R. G. Kathol and F. Petty, Relationship of Depression to Medical Illness: A Critical Review, *Journal of Affective Disorders, 3*, pp. 111-121, 1981.

89. F. K. Willits, R. C. Bealer, and D. M. Crider, Persistence of Rural/Urban Differences, in *Rural Society in the U.S.: Issues for the 1980s*, D. A. Dillman and D. J. Hobbs (eds.), Westview Press, 1982.

90. R. T. Coward and W. W. Smith, Jr., *Family Services: Issues and Opportunities in Contemporary Rural America*, University of Nebraska Press, Lincoln, 1983.
91. R. J. Scheidt, The Mental Health of the Aged in Rural Environment, in *The Elderly in Rural Society*, R. T. Coward and G. R. Lee (eds.), Springer Publishing Company, New York, 1985.

Chapter 9

SUBJECTIVE WELL-BEING AMONG THE RURAL ELDERLY POPULATION

Jay Meddin
and
Alan Vaux

This study is an investigation of the subjective well-being of the rural elderly population. A growing body of knowledge is developing that furthers our understanding of the subjective well-being of the general population of the United States [1, 2], and with this increase in understanding is a concomitant increase in interest in the subjective well-being of subcategories of the population such as the aged.

AGE VARIATION IN SUBJECTIVE WELL-BEING

We know that subjective well-being varies across the life span [3]; as students of life course have long observed, life experiences, subjective interpretations, and needs change as we move from young adulthood through the middle years and into older age [4]. The reasons for change are myriad and include social, psychological, and health factors.

From the social perspective, patterns of work, family life, and general social integration change systematically over the life span. For example, Blau has observed that friendship ties tend to be most important in adolescence and older age while nuclear family ties tend to be more important during the middle years [5]. From the personality perspective, life goals and perceptions of personal success also vary as one moves through the life course. To illustrate, Levinson found that for a sample of men, striving and establishing one's self were very important up to about the mid-forties; later, coming to terms with one's achievements and accepting them became more important than striving [6]. In regard to older populations, Campbell's survey data indicate that elderly persons (over 65) tend to be "more serene and less worried" than younger age groups [2, p. 176]. However, Campbell as well as others have found that satisfaction with health is one area that is an exception [3]. Not surprisingly, elderly people report less satisfaction with their health than do younger people.

Within the social environment, life changes influence individuals with varying frequency and intensity depending upon their location within the social structure [7], and clearly, age is one important factor in determining that location. In fact, the transition through the life span, until older age, can be viewed as a series of role entrances and exits [5], with concomitant changes in social resources (such as social support), psychological states, and health status.

SUBJECTIVE WELL-BEING AND ELDERLY PERSONS

Though well-being varies over the life span, it often does so in a manner that commonsense would not predict. As we indicated, findings show elderly persons to be generally more satisfied with their lives than other age groups [3], to worry less, except in regard to health [2], and to evidence less negative affect [8] and depression [9]. The stereotypes of older age as a period of decline in the quality of life do not hold up.

In speaking of elderly persons, as with any large social category, we must interject a note of caution, for they are a heterogeneous group. As Blau insightfully points out, structural factors such as education, ethnicity, employment, and marital status mediate the effects of age upon physical and mental health and self-conception [5]. In order to develop a more precise understanding of well-being among elderly persons, we need to focus upon particular aged populations and the psychosocial factors that influence their well-being.

As suggested by Blau's observations, there are a wide range of factors that might produce differences in subjective outlook and well-being among elderly persons. The rural elderly population is of particular interest, for the values of urban populations often differ by significant degree from those of the more traditional rural populations [10]. In this study, we focus on the rural elderly population, a category of elderly people that comprises over 28 percent of the elderly population of the United States [11].

Even though they comprise over 28 percent of the older population, we believe that rural elderly people are both understudied and underserved. We think it desirable to improve our knowledge base both in order to understand this segment of the older population better and to better ascertain their needs. In terms of emotional well-being, we want to know how rural elderly people differ from other elderly populations and how they are similar.

THE STUDY

The specific purpose of this study is to examine psychosocial influences on subjective well-being among a rural, elderly, midwestern population. The study employs multiple measures of well-being: specific and global, and positive and negative. The psychosocial influences include coping resources, social support, perceived physical well-being, life change, and income.

METHOD

Sample

Interviews were conducted with older adults at four senior citizens' nutrition and activity centers in four rural midwestern towns. One town had a population of 26,000 (some 70% of whom were students), while the remainder were considerably smaller (under 6,000). Previous research by Gunter on the aged in this geographic area indicated that persons attending these sites are representative of older people in their respective areas [12]. The median age of the study participants was seventy years. The sample was predominantly female (69%), white (81%), low income (median annual income was $7,000), nonworking (83%), and of low education (33% had reached grade 8 or less, 71% had reached grade 12 or less, and 40% did not have a high school diploma). Of the 140 interviews conducted, 100 provided complete data on all seventeen of the variables used in this study (many of which were multi-item scales), and analysis was restricted to these interviews.

Procedure

Structured interviews were conducted at the sites by the first author and three graduate students trained in interviewing and the use of the present instrument. Participants were carefully monitored for fatigue or loss of interest during the interviews. Very few interviews (less than 3%) were terminated prematurely.

Subjective Well-Being (Dependent Variables)

Seven indices of well-being were utilized in this study. Together these measures tapped the major components of well-being [8, 13]. Their selection was based on their demonstrated reliability and validity, and widespread use in community surveys of psychological well-being and quality of life [1, 2, 8, 14-16].

Positive Affect

Two measures tapping positive affect were used: Bradburn's five-item Positive Affect Scale taps the experience of five positive feelings during the previous few weeks [17], and has shown very good reliability and convergent and discriminant validity; a single item tapping current "happiness" was used that has shown good reliability and convergent validity [18].

Negative Affect

Two measures tapping negative affect were used: Bradburn's five-item Negative Affect Scale taps the experience of five negative feelings during the previous few weeks [17], and has demonstrated very good reliability and convergent and discriminant validity; a single item tapping the experience of "low spirits" has shown good reliability and convergent validity [18].

Composite Well-being

Several more global measures of well-being were used. The Centre for Epidemiological Studies Depression Scale (CESD) assesses both negative and positive affect to yield a measure of depressed mood. The twenty-item CESD has shown excellent internal consistency, good stability, and good convergent and discriminant validity [9, 19]. Dohrenwend et al. suggest that, like many similar measures, the CESD is best seen as a measure of "demoralization" when used with community samples [20]. Also used was a global satisfaction index, measuring satisfaction with major areas of respondents' lives: self, health, income, family, friends, town, and housing. The seven-item global satisfaction index was the sum of five-point satisfaction ratings ("not at all satisfied" to "extremely satisfied") with each of these areas. These items have been used widely in community surveys and have shown good psychometric properties [18]. A single-item was used to tap overall satisfaction with life; this item also has been used in community surveys and has shown good psychometric properties [18].

Psychosocial Variables (Independent Variables)

Life Events

An inventory of fifty-three life events was used. These events were drawn from previous research with community samples, especially the PERI [21], with the addition of items thought especially relevant to elderly people (e.g., overnight visits to friends or relatives). In addition, respondents could add life events they had experienced which were not listed. Few respondents added events, suggesting the relative completeness of the inventory. Participants indicated whether they had experienced the event during the past year. After reviewing classification of the same or similar items in previous research, the authors classified sixteen events as positive, twenty-eight as negative, and the remainder as ambiguous. Independent classification yielded virtually complete agreement. Further, of the forty events shared with the PERI, our classification of events as positive or negative showed 98 percent agreement with that of Dohrenwend et al. [21]. Positive and negative life event scores were computed as unweighted sums of items experienced within the last year.

Social Support

Two indices of social support were used here, focusing on support resources and perceived support respectively. First, support resources were represented by an index computed as the product of network size (the number of different persons providing four distinct kinds of social support), the frequency of contact with, and closeness to, network members [22]. Second, perceived support was assessed through a shortened (10-item) version of the twenty-three-item Social Support Appraisals Scale (SSA) [23]. Respondents rate statements such as "I am loved dearly by my family" and "I am held in high esteem" on a four-point agree-disagree scale. The SSA has shown excellent internal consistency and convergent validity in both students and community samples.

Coping Resources

Measures of three coping resources were used: a sense of mastery, low self denigration, and self-esteem. Pearlin and Schooler performed factor analysis of items thought to represent coping resources, resulting in these three measures [24] The scales have shown good reliability and validity [24].

Income, Age, and Perceived Health Problems

Finally, respondents provided data on their income, age, and perceived health problems. Income and age were recorded straightforwardly. Perceived health problems were assessed by the item "Do you have any problems with your health?"

RESULTS

In analysis we have posed four questions. First, which *specific* psychosocial factors are associated with which *specific* well-being variables? We have chosen to approach this question through bivariate correlation. Second, as a *set*, how well do the psychosocial variables correlate with the well-being variables as a *set*? Here we employ canonical correlation as the mode of analysis. Third, how well do the psychosocial factors predict each of the well-being variables? Fourth, which *particular* psychosocial factors stand out as important predictors of well-being? We seek to answer both these questions with multiple regression analysis.

Correlation between Specific Psychosocial and Well-being Variables

Correlations between the well-being and the psychosocial variables are presented in Table 1 (Panel A). In addition, correlations among well-being measures and among psychosocial factors are also presented in Table 1 (Panels B and C).

Table 1. Correlation of Well-Being and Psychosocial Variables[a]

Panel A: Well-Being with Psychosocial Variables

	Positive Affect	Happiness	Negative Affect	Low Spirits	Depressed Mood	Life Satisfaction	Global Satisfaction
1. Positive Events			-.11		-.13		
2. Negative Events				.17	.16	-.24*	-.31**
3. Mastery	.18*		-.42***	-.36***	-.45***	-.29**	.38***
4. Low Denigration	.23*		-.46***	-.42***	-.43***	-.13	.25*
5. Self-Esteem	.13			-.16		-.25**	.27**
6. Perceived Support	.21*	.11	-.32***	-.33***	-.29**	-.22*	.25**
7. Support Resources		.15			-.12	-.10	.15
8. Income	.12		-.19*	-.22*	-.17		.19*
9. Age	.12	.21*	-.26**	-.17			.19*
10. Health Problems		-.20*		-.21*		-.28**	-.40***

Panel B: Well-Being Variables

	1	2	3	4	5	6
1. Positive Affect	—					
2. Happiness	.49***	—				
3. Negative Affect	-.23*	-.29**	—			

	1	2	3	4	5	6	7	8	9
4. Low Spirits	-.31**	-.33***	.59***	—					
5. Depressed Mood	-.24*	-.15	.62***	-.47***	—				
6. Life Satisfaction	.18	.32***	-.38***	-.42***	-.32***	—			
7. Global Satisfaction	.31**	.33***	-.32***	-.34***	-.31**	.46***	—		

Panel C: Psychosocial Variables

	1	2	3	4	5	6	7	8	9
1. Positive Events	—								
2. Negative Events	.31**	—							
3. Mastery	.23*	-.23**	—						
4. Low Denigration	.17		.52***	—					
5. Self-Esteem	.18	-.31**	.12		—				
6. Perceived Support	.16	.16	.26**	.29**	.19*	—			
7. Support Resources	.19*	.10	.10	.33***			—		
8. Income		.11		.21*	-.17	.31**	.24*	—	
9. Age	-.17	.10		.21*					—
10. Health Problems		.13	.20		-.12		.20*	.22*	-.11

a Only those correlation coefficients exceeding .10 are included in the table.

* $p < .05$
** $p < .01$
*** $p < .001$

Panel A of Table 1 shows a number of statistically significant correlation coefficients; however, in the interest of space, only those coefficients at .30 or above are reported here. Negative life events correlates inversely at .31 with global satisfaction. Two of the more "psychological" resources, a sense of mastery and low self denigration, are moderately associated with a number of well-being measures. Both mastery and low denigration correlate inversely at greater than -.40 with negative affect and depressed mood. Low denigration correlates inversely at -.42 with low spirits, and in addition, mastery correlates inversely at above -.30 with low spirits[1] and positively with global satisfaction. Perceived social support (but not support resources) correlates inversely at greater than -.30 with negative affect and low spirits. Finally, perceived health problems and global satisfaction show an inverse correlation of -.40.

Positive life events show only a small negative correlation with negative affect and depressed mood. Income and age show small associations with most of the well-being variables and in the directions that one would expect.

Turning to the associations *among* well-being measures and psychosocial factors (Panel C), a number of relationships are worth mentioning; however, only the most notable are reported here. In Panel B, the correlations between negative affect and low spirits (.59) and negative affect and depressed mood (.62) stand out. In Panel C, the correlation between mastery and low denigration (.52) is worth noting (See Footnote [1] for further discussion of the relationship between these two variables.)

Canonical Correlation between Well-being and Psychosocial Variables

To get a global picture of these relationships, the association between the set of well-being measures and the set of psychosocial variables was examined through canonical correlation. The results are presented in Table 2. Only one canonical function was significant (canonical $r = .73$). Consonant with the previous findings, this function suggests a relationship largely between global satisfaction, low spirits, negative affect, depressed mood, and happiness on the one hand, and low denigration, mastery, perceived support, perceived health problems, negative life events, and income on the other. The canonical r is high, suggesting that the relationship between the sets of variables is strong.

Regression of Well-being Measures on Psychosocial Variables

How well do the psychosocial variables examined here predict each of the well-being indicators? In order to get a better understanding of the influence of psychosocial variables on the specific well-being indicators, separate regression analyses were performed with *each* well-being measure as the criterion variable.

---

[1]As we shall see in Panel C of Table 1, both mastery and low denigration are correlated with one another at above the .50 level. That they behave similarly in correlation with the negative well-being measures is hardly surprising.

Table 2. Canonical Correlation of Well-Being with Psychosocial Factors

Well-Being	Standard Canonical Coefficients	Psychosocial Factors	Standard Canonical Coefficients
Depressed Mood	.23	Income	−.26
Global Satisfaction	−.51	Age	−.10
Positive Affect	−.13	Health Problems	.22
Negative Affect	.25	Positive Events	−.09
Low Spirits	.39	Negative Events	.25
Happiness	−.28	Mastery	−.34
Life Satisfaction	−.04	Low Denigration	−.36
		Self-Esteem	.09
		Perceived Support	−.28
		Support Resources	.13

Canonical Correlation = .73
Wilk's Lambda = .24
Chi-Square (70) = 127.65***

*** $p < .001$

The results of these analyses are presented in Table 3. The psychosocial variables show significant relationships with five of the seven well-being measures. These variables account for about one-third of the variance in negative affect, low spirits, global satisfaction, and depressed mood, somewhat less in life satisfaction. Only about 10 percent of the variance could be explained in positive affect and happiness, and the regression equations were non-significant. Therefore, these latter results are not presented in Table 3, and positive affect and happiness are not discussed further.

Which specific psychosocial variables are important in predicting well-being? The findings are basically consistent with previous results. However, in answering this question, it is important to recognize that intercorrelations among the psychosocial variables might mask their predictive importance in the final regression equations. As suggested by previous findings, mastery, low denigration, and perceived health problems are statistically significant predictor variables. However, perceived social support drops slightly below the level of significance as a predictor (though its pattern of bivariate associations with well-being was noteworthy), and negative life events become significant.

Specifically, negative life events prodict global satisfaction. Mastery is a statistically significant predictor of both negative affect and depressed mood. Low

Table 3. Regression of Well-Being on Social and Psychological Variables

	Negative Affect		Low Spirits		Life Satisfaction		Global Satisfaction		Depressed Mood	
	β	F	β	F	β	F	β	F	β	F
Positive Events	.04	<1	—	—	—	—	—	—	-.04	<1
Negative Events	.03	<1	.12	1.47	.13	1.55	-.20	4.50*	.14	1.84
Mastery	-.24	4.18*	-.08	<1	.11	<1	.15	2.01	-.26	5.29*
Low Denigration	-.22	3.26	-.30	6.28*	.12	<1	.11	<1	-.21	3.03
Self-Esteem	-.04	<1	-.07	<1	.17	2.67	.13	1.89	-.10	1.15
Perceived Support	-.15	2.19	-.19	3.66	.13	1.50	.11	1.32	-.18	3.50
Support Resources	.11	1.36	.04	<1	.10	<1	.08	<1	.18	3.67
Income	-.10	1.04	-.10	1.00	.15	1.90	.07	<1	-.13	1.84
Age	-.19	3.52	.04	<1	.03	<1	.12	1.63	.05	<1
Health Problems	.04	<1	.16	2.81	-.24	5.38*	.32	12.09*	—	—
R^2	.33		.31		.23		.39		.33	
(d.f.) F	(10,88)	4.27**	(10,88)	4.01**	(10,88)	2.59**	(10,88)	5.53**	(9,89)	4.93**

* $p < .05$
** $p < .01$

140

denigration significantly predicts low spirits. Perceived health problems are a significant predictor of both life satisfaction and global satisfaction. Perceived social support predicts low spirits and depressed mood at a level of borderline significance. Variables that quite consistently contribute little to the prediction of well-being are positive life events, self-esteem, and income.

INTERPRETATION AND DISCUSSION

The results clearly indicate a relationship between well-being and variety of psychosocial variables. Canonical correlation analysis suggested that the relationship between well-being and psychosocial variables is quite strong. The regression analyses suggested that, with the exception of positive affect and happiness, indices of well-being are predicted by psychosocial variables. Mastery, low self denigration, perceived health problems, negative life events, and (less strongly) perceived support emerge as the psychosocial variables most consistently related to subjective well-being.

The profile that emerges for this sample of rural elderly respondents is quite consistent with the subjective well-being profiles both for the general and other elderly populations. The importance of mastery, nondenigration, social support, and perceived health status are readily interpretable on the basis of known literature.

The importance of efficacy and concomitant self-regard are themes that cut across clincal, community survey, and national survey literature. Bandura argues that enhanced efficacy is a major outcome of all successful counseling interventions [25]; Pearlin and Schooler (from whom the measures of mastery and nondenigration used in this study are derived) clearly demonstrated the importance of these variables in a large community study. In an extensive survey done in the Chicago area, mastery and nondenigration were found to be related to coping capacity and ultimately to subjective well-being. Campbell reports the findings of the Institute for Social Research's Quality of American Life national survey show that respondents with a strong sense of personal control also tend to report high levels of subjective well-being and satisfaction with self [2, 18].

The importance of mastery and nondenigration in subjective well-being persists across populations and age groups. The rural elderly population in this study are clearly no exception. These psychosocial factors are as important to their well-being as they are for others.

In general, health status tends to be an important issue for aged populations. As briefly mentioned at the beginning of this chapter, an extensive review and reanalysis of community and national surveys shows that a decline in health satisfaction seems to be one of the most important negative well-being relationships associated with age [3]. That perceptions of health is an important associative and predictive variable in this study is compatible with these findings. Perceived health status influences satisfaction for this rural elderly population just as it does for other elderly populations.

Social support universally is recognized as a major factor in emotional well-being [26]. Perceived support, though not support resources, showed a number of bivariate relationships with well-being, though these associations were attenuated by other predictors in the regression analyses. We think it noteworthy that it is *perceived* social support that is important and not support resources. Like so much of human affairs, social support is mediated cognitively, and the interpretation that we give to this resource has a major influence on its contribution to well-being. In regard to social support, as with mastery, nondenigration, and perceived health status, this sample of rural elderly persons seems similar to other populations.

The impact of life change varies with one's location in society and one's position in the life cycle [7]. In general, elderly persons experience fewer life changes that do younger populations, though these events tend to be more profound, e.g., death of a spouse or of friends. Although negative life events were significant in the prediction of global satisfaction, we find it surprising how little life events, negative or positive, contributed to subjective well-being in this analysis.

In conclusion, we find a moderate relationship between a wide range of well-being and psychosocial variables within this sample (note especially the canonical correlation findings). The influences on well-being among rural elderly people seem quite similar to those of other elderly populations, and to some degree, general populations. Factors such as a sense of mastery, nondenigration of self, health status, and social support, seem universal in contributing toward subjective well-being.

We think these findings worth noting. Though rural elderly persons comprise over 28 percent of the U. S. elderly population, comparatively less is known about their emotional well-being than urban elderly persons. To know that the same factors are associated with emotional well-being for both populations is useful. This information furthers our understanding of well-being among elderly people in general and helps us to understand well-being among rural elderly persons in particular.

REFERENCES

1. A. Campbell, P. Converse, and W. Rogers, *The Quality of American Life: Perceptions, Evaluations, and Satisfaction*, Russell Sage, New York, 1976.
2. A. Campbell, *The Sense of Well-Being in America*, McGraw-Hill, New York, 1981.
3. A. R. Herzog, W. Rogers, and J. Woodworth, *Subjective Well-Being among Different Age Groups*, Survey Research Center, Institute for Social Research, University of Michigan, Ann Arbor, Michigan, 1982.
4. R Linton, Age and Sex Categories, *American Sociological Review, 7*, pp. 589-603, 1942
5. Z. Blau, *Aging in a Changing Society*, Franklin Watts, New York, 1981.
6. D. Levinson, *The Seasons of a Man's Life*, Alfred Knopf, New York, 1978.
7. M. Tausig, Measuring Life Events, *Journal of Health and Social Behavior, 23*, pp. 52-64, 1982.

8. A. J. Zautra, Social Resources and Quality of Life, *American Journal of Community Psychology, 11*, pp. 275-290, 1983.

9. L. Radloff, The CES-D Scale: A Self-Report Depression Scale for Research in the General Population, *Applied Psychological Measurement, 1*, pp. 385-401, 1977.

10. L. Wirth, Urbanism As a Way of Life, in *Perspectives on the American Community,* R. Warren (ed.), Rand McNally, Chicago, Illinois, 1966.

11. R. C. Atchley, *Social Forces and Aging*, Wadsworth, Belmont, California, 1985.

12. P. Gunter, *A Survey of Needs of the Rural Elderly in Selected Counties in Southern Illinois,* unpublished doctoral dissertation, Southern Illinois University at Carbondale, Carbondale, Illinois, 1980.

13. F. M. Andrews and A. C. McKennel, Measures of Self-Reported Well-Being: Their Affective, Cognitive, and Other Components, *Social Indicators Research, 8,* pp. 127-155, 1980.

14. M. Block and A. J. Zautra, Satisfaction and Distress in a Community: A Test of the Effects of Life Events, *American Journal of Community Psychology, 9,* pp. 165-180, 1981.

15. L. Radloff, Sex Differences in Depression, *Sex Roles, 1,* pp. 249-265, 1975.

16. A. J. Zautra and L. Simons, Some Effects of Positive Life Events on Community Mental Health, *American Journal of Community Psychology, 7,* pp. 441-451, 1979.

17. N. Bradburn, *The Structure of Psychological Well-Being,* Aldine, Chicago, Illinois, 1969.

18. A. Campbell and P. Converse, *The Quality of American Life,* 1978, (machine readable data file), First ICPSR edition, Survey Research Center, Institute for Social Research, Ann Arbor, Michigan (producer), 1978; Inter University Consortium for Political and Social Research, Ann Arbor, Michigan (distributor), 1980.

19. L. Radloff, *Depression in Youth: Epidemic or Artifact,* paper presented at the American Psychological Association meeting in Washington, D.C., August 1982.

20. B. P. Dohrenwend, B. S. Dohrenwend, M. S. Gould, B. Link, R. Neugebauer, and R. Wunsch-Hitzig, *Mental Illness in the United States: Epidemiological Estimates,* Praeger, New York, 1980.

21. B. S. Dohrenwend, L. Krasnoff, A. R. Askenasy, and B. P. Dohrenwend, Exemplification of a Method for Scaling Life Events: The PERI Life Events Scale, *Journal of Health and Social Behavior, 19,* pp. 205-229, 1978.

22. A. Vaux and D. Harrison, Support Network Characteristics Associated with Support Satisfaction and Perceived Support, *American Journal of Community Psychology, 13,* pp. 245-268, 1985.

23. A. Vaux, J. Phillips, B. Thomson, L. Holly, D. Williams, and D. Stewart, The Social Support Appraisals (SSA) Scale: Studies of Reliability and Validity, *American Journal of Community Psychology,* in press.

24. L. I. Pearlin and C. Schooler, The Structure of Coping, *Journal of Health and Social Behavior, 19,* pp. 2-21, 1978.

25. A. Bandura, Self-Efficacy: Toward a Unifying Theory of Behavioral Change, *Psychological Review, 84,* pp. 191-215, 1977.

26. R. Leavy, Social Support and Psychological Disorder: A Review, *Journal of Community Psychology, 11,* pp. 3-21, 1983.

Chapter 10

SENIORS' ASSESSMENT OF THEIR HEALTH AND LIFE SATISFACTION: THE CASE FOR CONTEXTUAL EVALUATION

G. Elaine Stolar
Michael I. MacEntee
and
Patricia Hill

Professionals have been puzzled by seniors highly positive statements of their health and life satisfaction when compared with their own criteria-based ratings. In *Aging and Health Care,* Chappell, Strain, and Blandford review the current literature on health status and aging and summarize:

> . . . numerous surveys now exist that indicate a better subjective rating of health than would be assumed from the more objective measures of disease and disability [1, p. 39].

But, also:

> Diagnoses by physicians and self-reports may be highly correlated. These are similar to one another when individuals are asked about actual behavior rather than global questions about their health [1, p. 34].

There is considerable agreement with these statements [2-10]. One of the conclusions of the Canadian *General Social Survey, Health and Social Support, 1985,* is that the findings ". . . seems to suggest that people's aspirations change with age and that for most people their actual health is acceptable for the things they want to do" [11, p. 93].

Professional/researcher explanations for these evaluative differences center around assumptions that elderly individuals ignore their problems or that seniors use a cohort frame of reference. These ascribed frames include: life in older age is better than one had expected; is easier than youth and adulthood (was); and, I'm doing better than my peers (including, still being alive). Although there is anecdotal information that some individuals do make the above comments, there is little systematic evidence that they are explanations rather than assumptions. Structured survey data collection methods, the usual method employed to gather health and social information from seniors, is not designed to reveal respondents' frames of reference.

The positive correlations between self-evaluation of health and life satisfaction are important reflections of the quality of life. In fact, self-ratings of health have been shown to be good predictors of health status and mortality [12, 13]. It is acknowledged that the subjective response to a disease varies considerably, and there is increasing evidence that a positive response to stress can promote physical and emotional health [14-16].

North American theoretical models of aging have tended to reflect the social perceptions of growing old in a youth-oriented culture. After reviewing the literature, Connidis states that most aging materials fall into one of two categories: those that present a negative stereotype of aging, or those that present a positive stereotype [3]. Disengagement and low self-esteem were the focus of early research operationalized through measures of physical and mental health, losses of income, work, and significant others [17]. Activity theory, maintaining optimal levels of activity, is currently popular. In fact, "this view rests on extending the assumed virtues of youth, fitness, beauty, and sex into older age [3]. However, it is generally agreed today that no single standard can be used to determine the adequacy of activity patterns among mature adults [18].

Earlier authors developed a continuity theory of aging. For example, Clark and Anderson suggested that there is a set of adaptive tasks that aging persons have to deal with: recognition of aging and definition of instrumental limitations; redefinition of physical and social life space; substitution of alternate sources of need satisfaction; reassessment of criteria for evaluation of the self; and, reintegration of values and life goals [19]. They see the resolution of these demands as an interaction between personal development (one's self-image through time), and adaptation (learning to live with self and culture changes). Theirs is primarily a psychological approach.

An interactionist, Aaron Antonovsky specifically addresses health outcomes through the lifespan. He proposes that stressors are omnipresent and that stress may be salutary, contingent upon the character of the stressor and the successful resolution of the issue [20]. He calls this a salutogenic model of health which views health-sickness as a continuum along which every person moves. The approach ". . . leads us to reject the dichotomous classification of people as healthy or diseased in favor of their location on a multidimensional health ease/ disease continuum . . . (and) compels us to devote our energies to the formulation and advance of a theory of coping" [17, pp. 12-13]. To this end Antonovsky has developed the concept "Sense of Coherence" (SOC): a global orientation that expresses the extent to which one has a pervasive, enduring though dynamic feeling of confidence that stimuli deriving from one's internal and external environments are comprehensible, meaningful, and manageable [17, p. 19]. The SOC is developed over the lifespan and becomes ". . . a deeply rooted, stable dispositional orientation of a person" [17, p. 124].

As much research in aging has taken the form of surveys with closed response categories, there is little data available that allows understanding of the response-frame of older persons to questions regarding their life satisfaction and health status. The question is raised: Under what circumstances/conditions can one be satisfied with life and one's general health and, also, have decreases in functioning?

METHOD

Participants

This study is part of a larger study of general and oral health of community-dwelling seniors, seeking linkages between physical and social systems. The sample of 520 community-dwelling seniors was drawn from the list of voters of the City of Vancouver, B.C. To control for known age and sex discrepancies in the elder population, disproportionate stratified random-sampling procedures were applied to obtain equal representation for gender and age categories: seventy to seventy-four years, seventy-five to seventy-nine years, and eighty+ years. Of the 1600 persons contacted first by letter and then by phone, 489 persons were deceased, institutionalized, or had moved to an unknown address. Thirty-three were ineligible because of language, and 165 were too sick, leaving 915 eligible respondents. Of these, 43 percent refused participation and 57 percent completed the interview. At the time the project was beginning, a safety awareness program was directed toward seniors to deal with robberies and fraudulent strangers. It is likely this affected the response rate and is one possible explanation for the subsequent lower response rate of women. It is also likely that the sample is healthier than its population. Institutionalized elders were excluded from this sample and, therefore, the results apply only to community-dwelling seniors.

Procedures

The study was conducted between September, 1987 and June, 1988. Respondents were interviewed in their homes regarding their general and dental health, perceived health problems and attitudes, and their social support systems. The interviews were semi-structured and lasted an average of one hour, twenty minutes (Range = 45 minutes to 2 hours). Interviewers were trained to conduct the interview in a conversational mode and to record the spontaneous comments made pertaining to each question in addition to precoded response categories. All of those interviewed were offered an examination by a dentist, and 255 (49%) accepted.

The interview began with questions about current health, personal care, and health problems and moved to areas of life satisfaction and social networks. This article focuses on the self-reports of health and life satisfaction data.

To measure general health, individuals were asked: How would you describe your health right now? Is it excellent, good, fair, or poor? To measure oral health, individuals were asked: Would you say, in general, that your teeth or mouth are in excellent, good, poor, or fair condition? Adequate daily living functioning and common health complaints of seniors were queried to obtain more objective measures.

Several methods have been used to measure life satisfaction and well-being in a population, but the difficulty of scaling the data has led frequently to inconsistent results [21, 22]. The Life Satisfaction Index A of Neugarten, Havighurst, and Tobin, and adaptations, have been widely used [22]. In this study, the operationalization problem was addressed by asking the life satisfaction questions in a conversational mode and by recording the explanations and elaborations spontaneously framed by the respondents. The life satisfaction evaluation was tripartite: A) Thinking over your life **overall** would you say it has been: Very satisfactory, Average satisfaction, Not satisfactory; B) What about your life **now**? Very satisfactory, Average satisfaction, Not satisfactory; and, C) How do you feel about the **future**? Optimistic, Accepting, Pessimistic?

Percentage and frequency distributions were calculated on all questions. The chi-square statistic was used for bivariate analysis; level of significance set at $p < .05$. Content analysis was applied to the spontaneous comments made by the participants as they were answering the life satisfaction questions.

Description of the Sample

The sample is comprised of 51.9 percent males and 48.1 percent females. The mean age is 77.1 years; range 70 to 99 years. Seventy-five percent of the males are married, 15 percent are widowers, 4 percent are divorced and 6 percent never married. Thirty-four percent of the females are married; 51 percent are widowed, 4 percent are divorced and 11 percent never married.

Ninety percent of the respondents speak English in their homes; 62 percent were born in Canada, 16 percent in the British Isles; 52 percent were white collar workers before retirement (includes professionals), 17 percent housewives (never paid employment). Their median monthly income falls in the $1,000-$2,000 range currently and prior to retirement. Eighty-seven percent say their current income is adequate for their needs. In these respects, the sample is similar to other seniors in Canada [15].

All respondents make their homes in the community. Thirty-five percent live alone; 57 percent live with one other person. In this latter grouping, 97 percent of the co-inhabitants are over sixty-five years of age. Only 7 percent of the sample has a housing arrangement that involves more than one other person where at least one person is under sixty-five years.

Seventy-six percent of the respondents have living children. Almost 60 percent see their children once a week or more. There was no difference reported between male and female partners.

To offer a rough measure of social contact/isolation, respondents were asked: if they had left the house yesterday, 81.2 percent had; if they had talked to anyone on the phone yesterday, 77.3 percent had; and, if in the past week they had gone to any clubs or meeting, 41 percent had.

The profile of this sample is that they live alone or with one other contemporary, have children they see frequently, and they have regular social contacts.

RESULTS

Self-Evaluation of Health

Seventy-seven percent of the participants describe themselves to be in excellent or good general health. Oral health status was the only clinical data gathered in this study. Bivariate analysis of the self-evaluation of oral health contrasted with the clinical data. Generally the participants considered that their teeth and mouths were in good condition, three-quarters (78.1%) gave themselves a good or excellent rating, whereas the dentist estimated that only 13.4 percent of the mouths were healthy (Chi = 11.1; $df = 4$; $p = .02$). On the other hand, in response to the question, "Do you have any problem with your teeth, mouth, or dentures now?," there was a positive relationship with the dentist's observations (Chi = 5.7; $df = 2$; $p = .05$). These findings support the view that there is greater agreement between dentist and patient when the questions are focused to specific problems, as distinct from a more general self-assessment of oral health.

There is a very strong positive correlation between self-assessment of general health and the self-assessment of oral health (Chi = 100.7; $df = 9$; $p = .00001$). It is reasonable to assume, therefore, that the framework and/or assessment process used for general and oral health is similar in this age group.

Evaluation of Life Satisfaction

The expressions of life satisfaction in this sample were generally positive. Although more women were dissatisfied with their lives, both **Overall** and **Now**, and more men were pessimistic about the **Future**, the relationships between the measure of life satisfaction and age or gender was not significant (see Table 1).

All the participants who had Never Married reported satisfaction **Overall**, but they showed less satisfaction about **Now** and the **Future** compared to those who were or had been Married. Elders with children reported greater satisfaction **Overall** than those without children, but the presence of children did not contribute to current or future satisfaction.

Income is significantly associated with life satisfaction. As income increases so does life satisfaction: **Overall, Now and in the Future** ($p < .001$).

Over a quarter (29%) of the participants changed their **Overall** life satisfaction evaluation when addressing their current satisfaction, with 17.4 percent reporting they were less satisfied; 12 percent were more satisfied. An even larger proportion (40%) evaluate their life satisfaction **Now** differently than they foresee their **Future** life satisfaction: 18.5 percent expected things to improve and 21.2 percent expected a deterioration. On the other hand, about 54 percent of the respondents had a similar sense of satisfaction for all three time perspectives: 56.5 percent of the Very Satisfactory; 53.1 percent of the Average Satisfaction; and, 9.1 percent of the Not Satisfactory.

Content analysis was undertaken on the conversation between the respondent and the interviewers to obtain an indication of the meaning of the life satisfaction measures. Ninety percent of the sample made some comment but as the statements were spontaneous, not all participants are represented in each of the three categories. The analysis revealed that the participants in each response category used different language to describe their feelings, and they have been named accordingly: "the Optimists," "the Reconciled," and "the Disappointed" (Table 2).

A few gender distinctions were identifiable in these descriptions. For the Optimists, life satisfaction **Overall**: "Fun/Enjoyed" and "Good health" was all males; "Happy marriage" was all females. For life satisfaction **Now**: "Fewer responsibilities" was all females; "Retirement wonderful" was all males.

For the Reconciled, Life satisfaction **Now**: "Lonely" was predominantly females; "Better than before" was predominantly males. For life satisfaction

Table 1. Life Satisfaction Evaluation ($N = 520$)

	Thinking Over Your Life, How Would You Say:			
	It Has Been **Overall**	It is **Now**	You Feel About the **Future**	
Very satisfactory	53.4	49.6	48.4	(Optimistic)
Average satisfaction	44.3	45.1	45.0	(Accepting)
Not satisfactory	2.3	5.3	6.6	(Pessimistic)
	100.0	100.0	100.0	

regarding the **Future**: "Worry regarding finances" was all females. Generally the descriptors were not gender specific.

Examples of the language used by the participants is presented verbatim in Table 3.

Health and Life Satisfaction

All three life satisfaction measures were associated significantly with the self-assessments of health. High levels of life satisfaction are associated with high positive levels of health self-evaluation ($p < .001$).

Although there no independent measures of the respondents current health status, an attempt to determine adequate daily living functioning was made by asking: Does your health prevent you from doing some things for yourself? Climbing stairs, Moving about the house, Dressing, Bathing, Preparing meals, Eating meals? The only significant response related to life satisfaction was

Table 2. Descriptors[a] Accompanying Life-Satisfaction Rating
Ranked by Frequency of Response

	Optimists (Very Satisfactory)	Reconciled (Average Satisfaction)	Disappointed (Not Satisfactory)
Life **Overall**	Fun/Enjoyed Happy marriage Good health Lucky	Up & down Tough as a child Change some things Depressed/lonely	Hell as a child Disappointment Very sad life
Life **Now**	Happy Fewer responsibilities Retirement wonderful Family Healthy	Poor health (self or spouse) Making best of it Happy but . . . Decreased activity Lonely Better than before	Health problems Inactivity Lonely
Life in the **Future**	Life long optimist Faith in God Health concerns No choice	Just accept Day by day No choice Worry refinances Faith in God	State of world Fearful/unwell

[a]Descriptors were spontaneous, therefore not all participants are represented.

Table 3. Sample of Comments Accompanying Life-Satisfaction Responses

Life Overall:

Very Satisfactory
—F. 78 yrs: . . . except for the wars, life has been beautiful.
—M. 80 yrs: . . . heck of a lot of fun . . . everyone's been very nice to me
—F. 71 yrs: Wonderful! All the trouble has made me a better person
—M. 84 yrs: . . . perseverance . . . I've made a lot of myself

Average Satisfaction
—M. 76 yrs: . . . teenage was the worst time
—M. 81 yrs: We had a lot of trouble during the war but we survived and we're healthy
—F. 82 yrs: I'm a bit depressed . . . have travelled . . . lots of people . . . had to do it for myself
—F. 78 yrs: . . . would say it's better than it used to be

Not Satisfactory
—M. 75 yrs: . . . lot of disappointment . . . poor financial management . . . made good money . . . lost it all
—F. 85 yrs: . . . a life of hell when I was a youngster. I was a slave
—M. 75 yrs: . . . wild as a young man . . . didn't accomplish what could have
—F. 75 yrs: . . . hard as a child . . . broken home . . . foster child

Life Now:

Very Satisfactory
—F. 80 yrs: Now we are comfortable (financially) . . . more secure now than before
—F. 74 yrs: . : . own apartment . . . not poor . . . good health
—M. 78 yrs: When we're feeling good everything is great
—M. 76 yrs: . . . no punching clocks now . . . no money problems now

Average Satisfaction
—F. 72 yrs: It's rough going. My husband is very ill but we're managing
—M. 79 yrs: I'm not too happy about some things
—M. 78 yrs: The golden years are for the birds
—F. 80 yrs: I think we're treated so well compared to my grandmother

Not Satisfactory
—M. 75 yrs: . . . hard to not be active
—F. 71 yrs: . . . frustrating not being able to do things now
—M. 78 yrs: . . . health problems . . . the cancer . . . eye implants
—F. 82 yrs: . . . . I'm just existing, keeping going . . . my back . . .

Table 3. (Cont'd.)

Life in the Future:	Optimistic
	—M. 74 yrs: . . . that's my outlook . . . if things get bad they must get better . . . may take a while
	—M. 91 yrs: . . . better now than at any time in my life
	—F. 72 yrs: . . . so much I still want to do. If I knew how long I would live I'd spend every penny
	—F. 80 yrs: . . . hope the Lord will return real soon I want to go home . . . been blessed
	Accepting
	—M. 71 yrs: . . . apprehensive how long I'll last
	—F. 79 yrs: I've calmed down a lot
	—F. 79 yrs: I live one day at a time. I don't worry
	—M. 72 yrs: Good or bad you have to accept it
	Pessimistic
	—M. 73 yrs: . . . the world looks very shakey
	—M. 71 yrs: . . . for world . . . nuclear situation . . . all the injustice . . . military spending
	—F. 76 yrs: . . . world debt . . . monetary system . . . have lost so many of my family
	—F. 82 yrs: I'm lonely . . . believe in God which helps . . . don't have the disposition for solitude . . . no serenity

"difficulty climbing stairs." Participants were also asked if they had any problems with fifteen common health complaints of seniors (Table 4). A significant relationship was found between the life satisfaction measures and some "health" problems both **Now** and in the **Future**. The associated health problems appear to be predominantly functional disorders and/or problems which complicate daily functioning and social interaction. There are fewer health problems related significantly with **Future** life satisfaction (e.g., nervousness, sleeping, walking, seeing, eating and chewing, and hearing).

DISCUSSION

As in the case of previous studies, the self-assessment of health within this sample of elderly individuals was high compared to professional evaluations, and the measure of life satisfaction was higher than expected for individuals of this age.

Table 4. Distribution of Current Health Problems and Life Satisfaction **Now**:
Ranked in Order of Degree of Significance

| | Percent of Participants with Health Problem: Life Satisfaction **Now**: | | |
Health Problem	Very Satisfactory (%)	Average Satisfaction (%)	Not Satisfactory (%)
Nervousness*	17.7	31.1	54.2
Sleeping*	22.8	40.8	69.6
Walking*	26.2	36.7	60.9
Control of Bladder/Bowel*	14.5	17.1	45.5
Seeing*	24.7	32.2	56.5
Eating and chewing*	11.4	18.6	34.8
Kidneys and bladder*	11.5	16.7	36.4
Dizziness*	15.4	23.1	36.4
Heart trouble*	21.3	29.5	39.1
Remembering	47.0	57.8	47.8
Diabetes	5.2	8.6	4.5
High blood pressure	26.5	31.8	26.1
Hearing	35.4	40.2	43.5
Arthritis and rheumatism	48.5	51.7	58.3
Varicose veins	16.2	17.1	17.4

*$p < .05$

There is ample evidence in the literature that concerns about health are stressful, and that satisfaction is related closely to the subjective awareness and self-evaluation of health [3]. For the seniors in this study, some health problems were significantly related to current levels of life satisfaction. The Disappointed have most complaints, and the Reconciled have more than the optimists. The implications of ill health in this age group are complex. However, negatively associated with life satisfaction is a preponderance of functional disorders and/or problems which complicate daily functioning and interacting with others. The problems not significantly associated are chronic disorders with established treatments; more often they lend themselves to a greater sense of predictability and control, whereas the other group of disorders has more unknowns. For example, nervousness, not sleeping, being unsteady and/or pained on one's feet, all give feelings of apprehension and uncertainty. Frequently the "causes" of these problems are not singular, and sometimes unknown; further, the treatment may exacerbate the initial complaints. Arthritis and rheumatism, painful disorders, are a problem for over 50 percent of the respondents. Comparatively, the diagnosis is specific and the treatment regime established. A person knows what is happening to him/her; follows the prescribed regime (or not); and gets on with other aspects of living as best as s/he can. In Antonovsky's terms, the functional and interactional-stress disorders would make greater demands on one's sense of coherence.

It is important to keep in mind that health problems are present in all three levels of life satisfaction. The content analysis revealed that participants' evaluations were influenced by their past. Many references were made to war, the Great Depression, and radical social change; interpretations or evaluation of these events were distinctly different among the three groups:

- The Optimists express satisfaction and pleasure with their life, adding statements like: ". . . and we survived the depression"; ". . . trouble made me a better person." They turn stressors into strengths.
- The Reconciled usually began their comments on life with a reference to the stress they had to overcome and then moved to positives: ". . . life has been a struggle but we survived." Many references were made to war, depression and immigration. Several also made reference to having had a "tough life as a child."
- The Disappointed felt their life had been unsatisfactory, a disappointment, and they raised negative memories of childhood with statements like: ". . . hell as a youngster."

It appears that the three groups have different worldviews. The referents to childhood did not appear for the Optimists; the Reconciled use the word "tough," and the Disappointed use the word "hell." This suggests the above patterns did not arise in later life, but represent a long-standing response to stressors.

The movement by almost half (45.9%) of the participants emphasizes the importance of the framing and specificity of research questions. The three perspectives did elicit different responses quantitatively and qualitatively. The **Overall** measure appears to be an evaluation of the "whole" life; the **Now** measure a current and changeable evaluation; and, the **Future** a measure of expectations. Further, the three response categories present different attitudes: Life for the Optimists is "good"; for the Reconciled there is resignation, doing their best with the realistic demands of poor health (of self and/or spouse), economic insecurity, and loneliness; whereas, the Disappointed express a life out of control because of sickness, immobility, and loneliness.

This study supports the contention that health is related to life satisfaction and to an interpretation of the world. However, health-without-illness did not appear to be the comparative measure in this sample of elderly participants. Antonovsky's position that some stressors can be salutary when accompanied by a strong sense of coherence, and that coherence is "a stable dispositional orientation of a person" is supported [17]. The movement between the evaluations associated with the different timeframes indicates clearly that many older people do not experience or believe that growing old is necessarily "all down hill." This is not a denial of life's demands, but rather a frame of reference developed over a long life. Over half of the respondents consistently rated themselves in one life satisfaction category. From the comments given, there is evidence that movement between categories reflected a period of high stress, usually because of the exacerbation or resolution of illness, loneliness, or financial difficulties. That is, when one's internal and external environments are understandable, meaningful, and manageable, life satisfaction is positive. When these conditions are unstable, or are considered likely to become so, life satisfaction decreases. The application of different referents for different time perspectives is an important finding to be pursued by researchers and practitioners.

Intrinsically connected to "time" are the field(s) of experience out of which seniors respond to the questions of professionals. This study indicates that specific events, happenings and/or problems are not reliable indices of self-evaluation (overall) of health nor life satisfaction. Further research is required to determine to what extent seniors' and professionals' explanatory models of health are discrepant, thereby evoking miscommunication.

REFERENCES

1. N. L. Chappel, L. A. Strain, and A. A. Blandford, *Aging and Health Care: A Social Perspective,* Holt, Rinehart & Winston, Toronto, 1986.
2. W. R. Avant and P. L. Dressels, Perceiving Needs by Staff and Elderly Clients: The Impact of Training and Client Contact, *The Gerontologist, 20*:1, pp. 71-77, 1980.
3. I. Connidis, Life in Older Age: The View From the Top, in *Aging in Canada,* V. W. Marshall (ed.), Fitzhenry & Whiteside, Markham, Ontario, pp. 451-472, 1987.
4. I Connidis, The Subjective Experience of Aging: Correlates of Divergent Views, *Canadian Journal on Aging, 8,* pp. 7-18, 1989.
5. P. M. Keith, Evaluation of Services for the Aged by Professionals and the Elderly, *Social Service Review, 49,* pp. 271-278, 1975.
6. S. M. Kyriakos, Subjective Age, Health and Survivorship in Old Age, *Research on Aging, 4*:1, pp. 87-96, 1982.
7. G. R. Lee and M. Ishii-Kuntz, Special Interaction, Loneliness and Emotional Well-Being Among the Elderly, *Research on Aging, 9,* pp. 459-482, 1987.
8. V. W. Marshall, The Health of Very Old People as a Concern of Their Children, in *Aging in Canada,* V. W. Marshall (ed.), Fitzhenry & Whiteside, Markham, Ontario, pp. 473-488, 1987.
9. E. L. Snider, Explaining Life Satisfaction: It's the Elderly's Attitudes That Count, *Social Science Quarterly, 61*:2, pp. 253-277, 1980.
10. C. C. Wilson and F. E. Netting, Comparison of Self and Health Professionals' Rating of the Health of Community-Based Elderly, *International Journal of Aging and Human Development, 25*:1, pp. 11-25, 1987.
11. Government of Canada, *Health and Social Support, 1985,* Statistics Canada, Ottawa, Ontario, 1987.

12. J. M. Mossey and E. Shapiro, Self-Rated Health: A Predictor of Mortality among the Elderly, *American Journal of Public Health, 72*:8, pp. 800-807, 1982.
13. M. S. Goldstein, J. M. Seigal, and R. Boyer, Predicting Changes in Perceived Health Status, *American Journal of Public Health, 74*:6, pp. 611-614, 1984.
14. M. S. Gazzaniga, *Mind Matters,* Houghton-Mifflin, Boston, 1988.
15. B. Justice, *Who Gets Sick,* J. P. Torcher, Los Angeles, 1987.
16. E. L. Rossi, *The Psycho-biology of Mind-Body Healing,* Norton, New York, 1986.
17. A. S. Brown, *The Social Processes of Aging and Old Age,* Prentice-Hall, Englewood Cliffs, New Jersey, 1990.
18. R. C. Atchley, *The Social Forces in Later Life* (2nd Edition), Wadsworth, Belmont, California, 1977.
19. M. Clark and B. Anderson, *Culture and Aging,* C. C. Thomas, Springfield, Illinois, p. 214, 1967.
20. A. Antonovsky, *Unravelling the Mystery of Health,* Jossey-Bass, San Francisco, pp. 12-13, 124, 1987.
21. B. McKenzie and J. Campbell, Race, Socio-Economic Status, and the Subjective Well-Being of Older Americans, *International Journal of Aging and Human Development, 25*:1, pp. 43-61, 1987.
22. B. L. Neugarten, R. J. Havighurst, and S. S. Tobin, The Measure of Life Satisfaction, *Journal of Gerontology, 16,* pp. 134-143, 1961.

Chapter 11

EFFECTS OF BEREAVEMENT/LOSS AND PRE-EVENT STATUS ON SUBSEQUENT PHYSICAL HEALTH IN OLDER ADULTS

Stanley A. Murrell
Samuel Himmelfarb
and
James F. Phifer

A basic and broad assumption in psychosomatic research is that psychological stress can change physical health status. The high rate of research activity in the area of stressful life events is testimony to the potential significance for this basic assumption, although that research has shown generally weak effects [1, 2]. Among life events, deaths of significant others would appear to be the most intensely stressful, and therefore most likely to affect health. In this study, bereavement effects were studied in older adults for whom death is a particularly relevant event, since it can have severe economic, social, and psychological ramifications, and has been found to require more readjustment than any other stressful life event [3].

PREVIOUS RESEARCH

Research on Rates

Research on bereavement can be roughly grouped into four categories. Historically, the first of these involves the comparison of mortality *rates* of the widowed with those of the married using large national registers [4-6]. Kraus and Lilienfeld called attention to the fact that persons in the young (20 to 34 years) widowed group were about four times more likely to die of atherosclerotic heart disease and vascular lesions than were married people of the same age, as recorded by the U.S. Office of Vital Statistics [4]. Young et al. compared older married and widowers (55 and older) using a cohort identified from England's General Register Office, and found an increment of about 40 percent in deaths of the widowed within six months of their spouse's death [6].

Concurrent Comparisons

Another category of research compares a bereaved with a nonbereaved group. Bunch et al. observed that 50 percent of a group who had committed suicide had experienced a maternal death in the prior three years, compared to 20 percent in a matched control group [7]. Gallagher et al. found that their widowed group had higher distress but not greater serious psychopathology than a control group in an analysis that controlled for sociodemographic differences [8].

Follow-Up Studies

A third research category involves persons identified by the death of their spouse who are then followed over a period of time, with and without control groups. These studies, sometimes described as prospective studies, represent the most frequent type of research in this literature [e .g., 9-11]. Maddison and Viola interviewed widows and controls aged forty-live and older in Boston and Sydney about their health during the first thirteen months after the death of their spouse [9]. A higher proportion of widows had marked deterioration in health than controls, and Boston widows had more deterioration than Sydney widows. Parkes and Brown found that their bereaved group had higher hospital admissions in the year following their spouse's death than controls, and reported more symptoms related to the autonomic nervous system [10]. Thompson et al. followed a widowed group aged fifty-five to eighty-three for the two months after their spouse's death, and found them to have no greater number of hospital admissions or physician visits than a control group hut to be 1.4 times more likely to have a new or worsened illness, and 1.7 times more likely to have increased their use of medication [11].

Pre-Event Measurements

Overall, findings from research of these three types above would suggest that bereavement leads to a health decline. However, all three types share a methodological limitation: they have not measured and, therefore, cannot take into account the individual's health status prior to the bereavement. Thus, conditions related to prior health and to the death of the spouse may also lead to health changes in the survivor rather than the bereavement reaction itself. Only a few studies have been able to obtain measures on people prior to their bereavement experience. This allows prior status to be controlled, as well as avoiding the potential bias that may occur when subjects are knowingly chosen for the research because of a family member's death (i.e., a "guinea pig" effect). Heyman and Gianturco studied a subgroup of the Duke longitudinal sample (all 65 and older) who became widowed within a three-year period and found no changes in health after widowhood [12]. Helsing et al. examined the mortality rates with census type measures of a group eighteen years and older who became widowed within the eleven years following 1963 [13]. They found widowed males to have higher mortality than married males, but the rates were not different for females after an adjustment for a number of variables that also differentiated all widowed from all married (e.g., education, cigarette smoking, and percentage of time lived in housing with less than one full bathroom). Schleifer et al. compared lymphocyte responses in men before and after their wives had died of cancer, and found that lymphocyte stimulation was suppressed for two months following bereavement, which suggests a reduced immunity during the period [14]. Fenwick and Berressi studied lower income older adults (65 and older) who had changed their marital status during a fourteen-month period between interviews, and found that those who had lost a spouse had poorer perceived health, but also spent fewer days in bed than those who did not lose their spouse [15]. Moreover, it was the un-desirability of the event rather than the amount of change that the loss entailed that was important for health outcome.

EXPLANATIONS

Clayton, after a review of prospective studies, concluded that bereavement is a psychologically stressful event and is accompanied by psychological symptoms, but that within the first year men and women handle the event with minimal morbidity and mortality [16]. Generally, the better controlled studies show less of an effect on health. Here, we need to examine the possible reasons for an association between bereavement and health, and the methodological designs such studies would require.

Stress Reaction

One explanation is that the stress from the loss increases vulnerability to disease. Young et al. proposed that the "desolation effect" of being widowed was associated with changes in endocrine and central nervous systems, which would then reduce resistance to disease [6]. Klerman and Isen emphasized the disruption of attachment bonding in bereavement, and suggested mechanisms involving the hypothalamic and limbic systems and centers regulating neuroendocrine, sympathetic, and arousal functions [17]. Thus, the stress explanation does not target exclusive nor precise physiological mechanisms.

Homogamy

It is possible that people with poorer health tend to marry one another. Thus, the bereaved would have had poorer health prior to the death of their spouse compared to the nonbereaved [4].

Joint Unfavorable Environment

The likelihood that spouses, or relatives in general, have shared poor housing, unsanitary conditions, inadequate nutrition, inadequate medical services, etc., and that the bereaved survivor continues to be exposed to these conditions, suggests that the unfavorable environment that led to the family member's death may also contribute to higher morbidity and mortality of the survivor [4, 6].

The alternative explanations of homogamy and unfavorable environment would require that measures of health and environment be taken prior to the bereavement event. Then the question becomes: is it the event of bereavement itself that causes a decrement in health, apart from pre-event health and environment? That was the question for this study.

Compared to prior studies of this question, this study had these advantages:

1. it examined three different types of losses;
2. it included pre-event measures of health and environment;
3. it used multiple measures of health;
4. it used multiple measures of the impact of the event;
5. it used a large statewide community sample selected prior to the bereavement events; and
6. it examined both short-term and longer-term reactions.

METHOD

Sample

The sample for this study was from a larger longitudinal study of persons fifty-five and older who had been interviewed up to five times at six-month intervals. The longitudinal study used a stratified three-stage area probability design to select a statewide sample that reflected the three major geographic regions of Kentucky and several substrata within each region. This sample has been described in detail elsewhere [18, 19]. In general, the sample group was quite similar to the U.S. population in this age range in 1980 on its age and sex distributions, marital status, and living arrangements. However, the group had lower education levels. While two-thirds of the older adults in the U.S. census had more than an eighth-grade education, this was true for only one-half of this Kentucky sample [18].

Types of Bereavement/Loss

Respondents were selected from the larger sample if they had one or more events in three content categories of loss: *attachment bereavement*—a loss through death of a spouse, parent or child; *nonattachment bereavement*—a loss through death of a sibling, grandchild, or friend; *other losses*—the loss of a house, job, business, or pet, a decrease in money to live on; becoming separated or divorced; or having a child or a friend move away. Respondents were eligible for the present study only if they had a valid interview *prior* to the bereavement or loss event. In addition, a *no loss* group was included that had not experienced any of the above events *and* who had four consecutive interviews. The group assignment of respondents with events of more than one of these bereavement/ loss types was determined by these priorities: first—attachment bereavements; second—nonattachment bereavements; and third—other losses. If a respondent had the priority event at more than one wave, the earliest wave was used to maximize follow-up data for all but the no loss group. The "target" interviews for the no loss respondents were selected so that their distribution across waves was virtually the same as for the total bereavement/loss groups. The characteristics of this sample and the number of respondents in each bereavement/loss group are presented in Table 1. Of the total 1,572 respondents, 1,084 had four post-event interviews. The latter were thus available for five-wave analyses.

Physical Health Measures

Four of the five health measures were self-reports. This limitation was offset to some degree by measuring quite different aspects of health.

Health Status

This was a twenty-item self-report scale of symptoms, limitations of activity, and subjective evaluations of health that was adapted from one developed by Belloc et al. [20]. The scale has a possible range of scores from twenty to forty-nine, with a high score indicative of poor health. In the larger longitudinal sample, the scale had an internal reliability of .89 and a six-month test-retest correlation of .80. A preliminary validity study found that this scale discriminated between a subsample of the larger project sample and a matched "super healthy" sample of females not part of the project [21]. Health scale scores were significantly correlated with blood pressure, urinalysis indices, and twenty-one other biochemical measures.

Medical Conditions

Respondents were asked about the presence within the past year of ten medical conditions common to older persons (high blood pressure, nerves, kidney/bladder disease, heart trouble, serious lung trouble, stomach ulcers, cancer, hardening of the arteries, stroke, and diabetes). The variable used in the analyses was the

Table 1. Characteristics of Males and Females in the Sample

Wave A	Males		Females	
	Mean	SD	Mean	SD
Age	67.78	8.13	68.07	8.56
Education	9.05	4.42	9.48	3.81
Housing Quality	26.70	14.10	26.41	13.75
Service Availability	31.56	10.19	30.97	9.92
Health Status	30.94	7.38	31.74	7.18
Medical Conditions	1.68	1.70	1.67	1.60
Tenure (0 = Own)	.14	.35	.22	.41
Loss Group	N		N	
Attachment Bereavements	47		128	
Nonattachment Bereavement	463		718	
Other Losses	111		234	
No Losses	85		153	

number of these ten medical conditions reported. This variable had a test-retest reliability of .76 in the larger longitudinal study.

Death

This was the occurence of death at any point during the five wave project.

Medical Event

This was the report by the respondent of a "new illness or injury" in an interval between interviews.

Medical Services

Three items were used to estimate a need for medical services. These questions asked about the use of a hospital in the previous six months, seeing a physician in the previous six months, and whether the respondent was taking prescribed medication. The variable was the number of affirmative responses to these three questions.

Measures of the Environment

A number of measures were included to assess basic demographic variables and the nature of the respondents' physical and socioeconomic environment. *Age, sex, marital status* (married, widowed, separated, or divorced, and never married) were included in the analyses. Prior research suggested that geographic area might be relevant to health [22], so two dummy variables that indicated which of the three geographic *regions* (urban, rural, and Appalachian) of Kentucky in which the respondent resided were included. Because income information was not available on a large number of respondents, a number of other measures of socioeconomic status were included. These were: *education*—the number of years of schooling completed; *tenure*—whether or not the respondent owned or rented his/her housing; and *housing quality*—a measure of housing quality based upon the interviewer's rating of the external appearance and condition of eight aspects of the dwelling unit. The scale was scored so that a high score was indicative of poor housing. The internal consistency of the housing quality measure items was .97 in the larger longitudinal study. In addition, a *services availability* variable was included that assessed the availability of health and social services in the area in which the respondent resided. This measure was based on results of a previous needs assessment in which about 200 telephone interviews, on average, were conducted in each of fifteen geographic districts encompassing the entire state [23]. For the measure used here, the fifteen districts were ordered according to the toltal percentage of respondents in that district who rated seven social or medical services as "difficult to get" or "not available at all." The score for those in the present sample was that percentage for the district in which the respondent lived with a high score indicative of poor service availability.

Event Impact Measures

The Louisville Older Persons Event Scale was developed and pretested on earlier sample of older adults [24]. It included fifty-four closed-ended and two open-ended events. Respondents were asked whether each of the events had occurred in the prior six months and, if so, were asked to respond to five probes about the event. Further details on the development and pretesting of this instrument are available elsewhere [25], and data on the annual frequencies of each of the events and their mean desirability ratings for males and females in the larger longitudinal sample are also available [24]. Four event measures were derived from this scale and its probes, as described below, and were used in the analyses to assess the impact of the three event categories on physical health.

Number of Events

This measure was a simple count of the number of events in that category for that measurement wave. For both attachment and nonattachment bereavements these scores could range from zero to three and for the other losses category could range from zero to seven. (There were 8 events in the other losses category but 2 events, divorce and marital separation, were mutually exclusive.)

Change

For each event that had occurred, the respondent was asked to rate how much change in usual activities the event produced from one (almost no change) to four (large amount of change). The score within each event category was the sum of these ratings of the events in that category. These scores could range from zero to twelve for the two bereavement categories and from zero to twenty-eight in the other losses category.

Undesirability

For each event that had occurred, the respondent also was asked to evaluate the change produced by the event from -3 (very bad) to +3 (very good). The score within each category was the sum of the ratings of the events in that category. Theoretically, the scores in the two bereavement categories could range from -9 to +9 and from -21 to +21 in the other losses category. However, only a few of these events were ever rated positively.

Preoccupation

For each event that had occurred, the respondent was asked further to rate how much it was on his/her mind from one (very seldom) to four (very often). The score within each category was the sum of the ratings of the events in that category and the range of possible scores were the same as for the *change* measure.

For each of the four event impact measures, respondents could have a score in each of the three event categories if they had experienced events in the attachment bereavement, nonattachment bereavement, and other losses categories on a given measurement wave. If respondents had no events in a category, they received a score of zero for all impact measures for that content category. Respondents in the no losses group had zero scores in all three content categories on all four impact measures. A high score on *number of events, change,* and *preoccupation* indicated more events, more change, and more preoccupation, while a low score (more negative) on undersirability indicated more undesirability of events in that category.

RESULTS

All respondents had at least two interviews with a six-month interval between the two interviews. The interview *before* the event is designated wave A and the interview *after* the event is wave B.

Prior Health-Environment Factors and Subsequent Events

Table 2 presents the Pearson correlation coefficients between prior health status, medical conditions, and environmental variables on wave A, and the

Table 2. Correlations between Prior Health and Environmental Variables
and Subsequent Number of Attachment Bereavements,
Nonattachment Bereavements, and Other Losses

	Males (N = 523)			Females (N = 952)		
Variables	Attach-ment	Nonattach-ment	Other Losses	Attach-ment	Nonattach-ment	Other Losses
Health Status	-.009	.009	.026	.024	.066*	.048
Medical Conditions	-.083	.029	-.012	.034	.043	.057
Age	.057	.155***	-.200***	-.001	.086**	-.131***
MS1 (Married)	.031	-.029	-.006	.126***	-.098**	.017
MS2 (Widowed)	-.023	.048	-.042	-.087**	.108***	-.040
MS3 (Sep./Div.)	-.023	.025	.085	-.026	-.020	.042
Region 1 (Urban)	.108*	-.054	.092*	.044	-.086**	-.004
Region 2 (Rural)	-.046	.034	.018	-.026	.093**	-.004
Education	.011	.023	.081	.007	-.012	-.042
Tenure	.003	.046	-.004	.019	-.013	.015
Housing Quality	-.034	-.046	.012	.054	-.026	.077*
Service Availability	-.066	-.088*	-.094*	-.044	-.049	-.059

*$p < .05$.
**$p < .01$.
***$p < .001$.

number of events in each event content category within the wave A-B interval
as reported on wave B. Table 2 shows that one's status prior to the bereavement or
loss events is correlated with those subsequent events. For both males and
females, the older a person was at wave A, the greater the likelihood of experiencing more subsequent nonattachment bereavements (death of sibling, grandchild,
or friend) and the less the likelihood of losses other than bereavement. For
females, poor health, nonmarried marital status (i.e., widowed, divorced/separated,
or never married), and less urbanized residency also were significantly correlated
with nonattachment bereavements. As might be expected, married females at
wave A were more likely to experience attachment bereavements (death of
spouse, parent, or child), and widowed females less likely to experience a similar
loss. Females with poor housing were more likely to experience nonbereavement
losses. Males who resided in a more urbanized region experienced more attachment bereavements and more nonbereavement losses. Males who lived where
available social and medical services were poor tended to have fewer nonattachment bereavements and other losses.

Similar patterns of relationships were obtained when other event impact
measures were correlated with these prior status variables. Indeed, the relationships were often stronger when the impact of the events was measured by change
or undesirability. Of particular interest are the correlations between prior health

status and medical conditions and subsequent event impact scores. For both males and females, poor health—either as measured by the scale or a count of medical-conditions—was significantly associated with greater undesirability of nonattachment bereavements and other losses.

Although these relationships are quite modest, they do need to be considered in assessing the impact of bereavement and other loss events on subsequent physical health. These prior status variables are confounded with these events and unless they are taken into account, analysis of the effects of these events on subsequent health could yield spurious relationships or overestimates of the effects of the events on health.

Short-Term Effects of Events on Health

A series of multiple-regression analyses were conducted using either health status or medical condition scores at wave B as the dependent measure. The four event impact measures (i.e., change, undesirability, etc.) were separately analyzed. Scores in the three bereavement/loss categories (i.e., attachment bereavement, nonattachment bereavement, etc.) were considered simultaneously in each analysis. The regressions were performed hierarchically with the environment variables of wave A entered first, then the event impact scores for the three content categories obtained at wave B for the prior six months, and then the health measure for wave A (either the health status or medical conditions variable corresponding to whichever of the two was the dependent measure). This allows a comparison of the effects of bereavement/loss on health before controlling for pre-event health with that of the effects of events after such control. Then interaction terms of the event measures with the health measure on wave A and with each of the environmental measures were entered.

Table 3 reports the R^2 change that each set of measures contributed for males and females separately, for each event impact measure, for health status and for medical conditions. The environmental set made small but significant contributions to both health measures for all combinations. The bereavement/ loss event set also made significant contributions before the wave A health measure was entered for all combinations except three: number of events for males for both health measures and change for females on medical conditions. The wave A health measure made strong and significant contributions for both wave B health measures and for all combinations, with increases in R^2 that ranged from .439 to .483. The set of interaction terms did not make a significant contribution in any of these analyses. Essentially the same pattern was found for each event impact measure.

To compare the contribution of bereavement/loss events before and after pre-event health was entered, Table 4 reports the event betas for each type of bereavement/loss for each sex and each health measure for the four event impact measures. There were eighteen significant betas before health was entered and

Table 3. R² Changes for the Set of Environmental, Bereavement/Loss, Health, and Interaction Measures for Males and Females in Predicting Subsequent Health

Set of Measures	Males				Females			
	Change	Undesir-ability	Pre-occupation	Number of Events	Change	Undesir-ability	Pre-occupation	Number of Events
Health Status								
Environmental	.268***	.268***	.268***	.268***	.193***	.196***	.191***	.193***
Bereavement/Loss Groups	.020**	.011*	.021**	.008	.012**	.018***	.011**	.006*
Health on A	.447***	.455***	.445***	.456***	.483***	.472***	.484***	.487***
Interactions	.014	.013	.015	.019	.007	.006	.007	.007
Multiple R	.87	.87	.87	.87	.83	.83	.83	.83
df	41/486	40/484	40/485	40/486	40/928	40/918	40/925	40/928
Medical Conditions								
Environmental	.173***	.174***	.174***	.173***	.109***	.110***	.109***	.109***
Bereavement/Loss Groups	.018**	.018**	.014*	.005	.005	.014*	.006	.003
Health on A	.440***	.441***	.442***	.450***	.448***	.439***	.448***	.450***
Interactions	.023	.024	.028*	.020	.015	.012	.014	.014
Multiple R	.81	.81	.81	.80	.76	.76	.76	.76
df	41/496	40/493	40/493	40/496	40/933	40/921	40/930	40/933

* $p < .05$.
** $p < .01$.
*** $p < .001$.

169

Table 4. Betas for Bereavement/Loss Measures
Before and After Pre-Event Health Was Entered

| | Health Status | | | | Medical Conditions | | | |
| | Males | | Females | | Males | | Females | |
Independent Variables	Beta Before Health	Beta After Health	Beta Before Health	Beta After Health	Beta Before Health	Beta After Health	Beta Before Health	Beta After Health
Change								
Attachment	.016	-.024	.037	.012	.024	.053*	.041	.009
Nonattachment	.100**	.032	.052	-.008	.070	.026	.026	-.016
Losses	.123**	.037	.104***	.042*	.131***	.063*	.067*	.013
R	.536	.857	.452	.829	.437	.794	.338	.750
Undesirability								
Attachment	-.005	.029	-.052	-.026	-.023	-.052	-.068*	-.016
Nonattachment	-.046	-.012	-.065*	-.007	-.003	.016	-.051	-.007
Losses	-.100**	-.031	-.118***	-.046*	-.134***	-.063*	-.090**	-.030
R	.529	.857	.463	.828	.438	.795	.352	.750
Number of Events								
Attachment	.008	-.024	.025	.003	-.001	.038	.030	-.006
Nonattachment	.056	.000	.051	-.016	.001	-.030	.033	-.001
Losses	.093*	.012	.082**	.032	.074	.017	.053	-.017
R	.526	.856	.447	.829	.421	.792	.335	.750
Preoccupation								
Attachment	.027	-.015	.041	.011	.027	.052	.038	.003
Nonattachment	.086*	.016	.073*	-.001	.025	-.011	.057	.002
Losses	.138***	.038	.090**	.038*	.120**	.043	.061	.012
R	.538	.857	.449	.828	.433	.793	.338	.750

* $p < .05$.
** $p < .01$.
*** $p < .001$.

only six after health was entered. Of these six, five were for loss events, one for attachment bereavements; three were for males and three for females; three were for health status and three for medical conditions; three were on the change impact measure, two were on undesirability, one for preoccupation, and none for number of events. Thus, the overall picture suggests a slight impact when prior health is controlled and that impact is primarily from losses other than bereavements.

To compare the contributions of the various environmental influences on wave B health, Table 5 reports the betas for the environmental measures for each sex and for the health status and medical condition dependent variables from the regression equations after the corresponding wave A health measure had been entered. These values were from analyses that used the undesirability event impact measure; however, the results were very similar regardless of the event measure used. Table 5 shows a significant negative beta for education that indicates that the higher the number of years of education the better the person's health status on wave B. Thus, education made a significant contribution to health status at wave B for both sexes even with wave A health status partialled out, but contributions to medical conditions were not significant. Services availability made a significant contribution for both dependent measures, but only for females. Thus, some environmental variables appear to make an independent contribution to certain aspects of health on wave B that are not mediated by their effects through physical health on wave A or their effects through subsequent bereavement or loss events.

Death Following Bereavement/Loss

In this analysis, death was the dependent measure. The intent was to determine whether the proportion of deaths in the bereavement/loss groups (subsequent to the event) would be higher than that in the no loss group. Deaths were as reported by interviewers when they attempted interviews. An additional category here was "missing" which was the designation given respondents who were not interviewed on some interview wave because they could not be located nor could it be

Table 5. Betas for Pre-Event Environmental Influences on
Subsequent Health with Prior Health and Undesirable Impact
of Bereavement/Loss Partialled

	Males		Females	
	Health Status	Medical Conditions	Health Status	Medical Conditions
Education	.089**	.059	-.070***	-.029
Tenure	.031	.022	.000	.000
Services Availability	.035	.045	.081*	.117**
Housing Quality	.013	.032	.027	.016
Urban Region (1)	-.037	-.035	.047	.096
Urban Region (2)	-.023	.025	.000	.042

* $p < .05$.
** $p < .01$.
*** $p < .001$.

determined that they had moved. Since some of these respondents may well have died (or had a incapacitating health problem), they were included here. On the possibility that an accumulation of bereavement/losses would increase the death rate, respondents also were grouped together who had had two or even all three of the types of losses in one six month interval. The findings are reported in Table 6. As that table shows, having bereavements or other loss events did not lead to a higher probability of death.

Medical Events Following Bereavement/Loss

Here the question was whether bereavement/losses would be related to subsequent increases in reports of new illnesses or new injuries by the respondents. A discriminant function analysis was performed with occurrence versus nonoccurrence of a medical event as the dependent variable. The independent measures were the same as those in the regression analyses and their sequence of entry was the same. As before, prior health was by far the strongest predictor of medical events. The bereavement/loss set of measures made a significant contribution for females ($F = 1.73$, $p < .05$), but not for males before health was entered. After health was taken into account neither was significant. However, here a significant

Table 6. Comparisons on Percentages of Subsequent Deaths and Missing Interviews in Bereavement/Loss Groups with the No Loss Group

Group	N	Died (Percent)	Missed Some Interviews (Percent)	Completed All Five Interviews (Percent)	x^2
No Loss	1774	4.1	52.5	43.4	
Attachment Bereavement	46	0.0	58.7	41.3	2.24
Nonattachment Bereavement	563	2.8	51.3	45.8	2.36
Other Losses Only	328	2.1	50.6	47.3	3.86
All Three Losses	3	0.0	0.0	100.0	3.90-
Attachment and Nonattachment	13	7.7	38.5	53.8	1.22
Attachment and Other Losses	22	4.5	40.9	54.5	1.19
Nonattachment and Other Losses	182	3.8	50.5	45.6	0.32

Note: None of the analyses yielded significant x^2 values.

interaction was found for health by the set of bereavement/loss measures for both males ($F = 1.91$, $p < .05$) and females ($F = 2.22$, $p < .01$). The direction of this interaction was examined, and it indicated that increased medical events were most likely when bereavement/losses occurred to those in better health, which was an unexpected pattern.

Medical Services

The measure of medical services was an index involving three items: whether or not a doctor's care for a medical problem had been needed in the past six months, whether or not hospital care for a medical problem had been needed, and whether or not medicine prescribed by a doctor was being taken. The index was an unweighted score that correlated .46 with health status and .54 with medical conditions (for both, $p < .001$). Since these services were not dated within the prior six-month interval, there was no way to insure that the bereavement/loss event occurred before the medical service usage if the wave B measure was used. Therefore, the wave C measure of medical services was used, which meant that these medical services were used between one month to eleven months later, depending on when the bereavement/loss event and the medical service usage occurred. Neither the environmental variables nor tbe bereavement/loss events made a significant contribution even before wave A medical services and health were entered and did not do so afterward. Thus, bereavement/loss events were not related to increased use of medical services.

Longer-Term Effects of Bereavement/Loss Events

In order to determine possible longer-term effects of bereavements/losses on health over time, multiple-regression analyses of the trend over wave A to wave E were conducted. The dependent variables for these analyses were the linear, quadratic, cubic, and quartic trend components, obtained by multiplying the wave A through E health status scale scores by the appropriate orthogonal polynomial coefficients and summed across waves. As in the previous analyses, the predictor variables were organized into hierarchical blocks and entered in the following order: environmental variables, bereavement/loss event scores, two-way, and then three-way interaction terms. For the analyses of higher order trend components, the lower order trend scores were entered also (prior to the interaction terms). The event impact scores used in these analyses were the number of events and change.

In the linear trend analyses for both impact measures, attachment bereavements (number of events beta = -.07, change beta = -.06, $p < .05$) and other losses (number of events beta = -.10, change beta = -.11, $p < .05$) yielded an *improvement* in health status across waves A through E. Also, both impact measures yielded significant quadratic trends for other losses (number of events and change beta = -.091, $p < .05$). None of the other components was significant. The negative betas of the quadratic component for other loss events indicate an inverted U-shaped relationship over time. Because higher health scores were indicative of poor health, this trend shows a worsening of health followed by subsequent improvement over time. The decrease in health for other losses is consistent with the short-term results reported under the wave B analyses. The negative linear trend for other losses indicates that the later improvement was much greater than the initial decrease in health. For attachment bereavements, there was only a linear trend indicative of improved health over time. None of the trend components was significant for nonattachment bereavements.

DISCUSSION

Consistent with Clayton's review conclusions, this older adult sample handled bereavements and other losses with minimal morbidity and mortality [16]. Using a variety of health indicators, the effects of these events were either nonexistent or slight and brief. In fact, health improved over the long term following bereavement.

Among the event, environmental, and health variables considered, this study found that the best predictor of the physical health of an older adult at any given point in time clearly is the person's previous health. Moreover, because of the strong relationships obtained between prior and subsequent health, any claims of the effects of bereavements/loss on subsequent health must be viewed with extreme care and, perhaps, suspicion. Differences that have been obtained may reflect prior health status rather than subsequent consequences. For the present sample, prior health status was correlated with later experiences of nonattachment bereavements and other losses. Although attachment bereavement was not significantly related to prior health, the two were positively correlated. Also, it was significantly correlated with some environmental factors.

The environmental factors considered in this study also made consistent significant contributions to health (particularly education) prior to considering pre-event health. After the inclusion of previous health, instances of significant contributions remained but they were much reduced. Environmental variables did not predict attachment bereavements, but there were significant predictors of nonattachment bereavements and other losses. While not particularly strong, there did appear to be some relationship between environmental factors and health, both directly and indirectly through bereavement/losses. Thus, the hypothesis that a joint unfavorable environment might be responsible for an association between bereavement/loss and subsequent health does receive rather modest support in the present study.

This study examined three types of losses: attachment bereavement, nonattachment bereavement, and other losses. It was expected that if these events had an effect on physical health, attachment bereavements would have the most severe effects and other losses the least strong affects. However, the results showed the opposite pattern. Of the three types of events, other losses showed the strongest effects on health, albeit modest and reduced ones, on wave B when prior health was accounted for in the regression equations. In the wave A through wave E trend analyses, other losses were associated with a decline followed by a more rapid increase in health. Thus, these three types of losses appear to have different relationships to health prior and subsequent to the events, although in ways contrary to expectations and common belief.

One possible explanation for the stronger effect of other losses is that the category may have contained more events that were less anticipated (e.g., loss of job or house) for this age group than death. Having less preparation for them may have led to their greater impact. Another possible explanation is that of restricted range. The other losses category did have a greater potential range of scores than either of the two bereavement categories. However, the use of event impact measures (change, undesirability, preoccupation) in addition to just the number of events was intended to make up for some of this disparity. In addition, the number of people who experienced events in each category differed markedly. For example, only 175 respondents in the wave A-B analyses had an attachment bereavement, while 1181 respondents had a nonattachment bereavement. Nonetheless, this number of cases in the attachment bereavement group was still sizeable in comparison to many other studies of bereavement in the literature. Moreover, the inclusion of persons within other categories of losses and with no losses in the same analyses increased the power of the study to detect small differences. Yet, no effects of attachment bereavements on subsequent health were found regardless of whether health was measured by the health status scale, medical conditions, mortality, the seeking of medical services, or the experience of a new illness or injury.

It is also important to note that in the longer term analyses, the sample's health actually improved following attachment bereavements and other losses. Perhaps the wave A health was being affected by factors related to the impending event. When the event occurred and those factors diminished, health may have then returned to its pre-wave A level.

Given the pattern of relationships found here, extreme caution in interpretation is necessary especially since controlled experiments are impossible to conduct. What is often considered a control group may be a group that is matched on, at the most, only a few variables. Consistency of findings in the area will be difficult to obtain given the present variability among studies in the types of designs, measures, and kinds of variables that are considered as dependent, independent, and control variables. Given these limitations and cautions, the best conclusion from the present data is that we were unable to detect any detrimental effects of bereavements on physical health, although other losses did have small and transient effects. Since some of these other losses (e.g., loss of home, job, or business; child move away) alter the environment and the resources people have available to them, the results are not inconsistent with an environmental explanation for changes in physical health.

REFERENCES

1. S. Cobb, A Model for Life Events and Their Consequences, in *Stress and Life Events: Their Nature and Effects*, B. S. Dohrenwend and B. P. Dohrenwend (eds.), Wiley, New York, 1974.
2. J. G. Rabkin and E. L. Struening, Life Events, Stress and Illness, *Science, 194*, pp. 1013-1020, 1976.
3. D. Gallagher, L. W. Thompson, and J. A. Peterson, Psychosocial Factors Affecting Adaptation to Bereavement in the Elderly, *International Journal of Aging and Human Development, 14*, pp. 79-95, 1981-82.
4. A. S. Kraus and A. M. Lilienfeld, Some Epidemiologic Aspects of the High Mortality Rate in the Young Widowed Group, *Journal of Chronic Diseases, 10*, pp. 207-217, 1959.
5. S. A. Melstrom, A. Nilson, A. Oden, A. Rundgren, and A. Svanborg, Mortality Among the Widowed in Sweden, *Scandanavian Journal of Social Medicine, 10*, pp. 33-41, 1982.
6. M. Young, B. Benjamin, and W. Wallis, The Mortality of Widowers, *Lancet, 2*, pp. 454-456, 1963.
7. J. Bunch, B. Barraclough, B. Nelson, and P. Sainsbury, Suicide Following Death of Parents, *Social Psychiatry, 6*, pp. 191-193, 1971.
8. D. E. Gallagher, J. N. Breckenridge, N. James, L. W. Thompson, and J. A. Peterson, Effects of Bereavement on Indicators of Mental Health in Elderly Widows and Widowers, *Journal of Gerontology, 38,* pp. 565-571, 1983.
9. D. Maddison and A. Viola, The Health of Widows in the Year Following Bereavement, *Journal of Psychosomatic Research, 12*, pp. 297-306, 1968.
10. C. Parkes and R. Brown, Health After Bereavement: A Controlled Study of Young Boston Widows and Widowers, *Psychosomatic Medicine, 34*, pp. 449-461, 1972.
11. L. W. Thompson, J. N. Breckenridge, D. Gallagher, and J. Peterson, Effects of Bereavement on Self-Perceptions of Physical Health in Elderly Widows and Widowers, *Journal of Gerontology, 39,* pp. 309-314, 1984.
12. D. Heyman and D. Gianturco, Long-Term Adaptation by the Elderly to Bereavement, *Journal of Gerontology, 38,* pp. 259-362, 1973.
13. K. Helsing, M. Szklo, and G. Comstock, Factors Associated with Mortality After Widowhood, *American Journal of Public Health, 71,* pp. 802-809, 1981.
14. S. J. Schleifer, S. E. Keller, M. Camerino, J. C. Thornton, and M. Stein, Suppression of Lymphocyte Stimulation Following Bereavement, *Journal of the American Medical Association, 250,* pp. 374-377, 1983.
15. R. Fenwick and C. M. Barresi, Health Consequences of Marital-Status Change Among the Elderly: A Comparison of Cross-Sectional and Longitudinal Analyses, *Journal of Health and Social Behavior, 22*, pp. 106-116, 1981.
16. P. J. Clayton, The Sequelae and Nonsequelae of Conjugal Bereavement, *American Journal of Psychiatry, 136,* pp. 1530-1534, 1979.
17. G. Klerman and J. Izen, The Effects of Bereavement and Grief on Physical Health and General Well Being, *Advances in Psychosomatic Medicine, 9*, pp. 63-104, 1977.
18. S. A. Murrell, S. Himmelfarb, and K. Wright, Prevalence of Depression and Its Correlates in Older Adults, *American Journal of Epidemiology, 117*, pp. 173-185, 1983.

19. G. S. Bonham and R. M. Savage, *Sampling and Weighting Procedures: Resources, Stress, and Mental Health of Older Persons*, Working Paper No. 19, Grant No. MH33063, University of Louisville, Urban Studies Center, Louisville, Kentucky, 1983.

20. N. Belloc, L. Breslow, and J. Hochstim, Measurement of Physical Health in General Population Surveys, *American Journal of Epidemiology, 91*, pp. 105-111, 1971.

21. A. F. Brennan and S. A. Murrell, *Establishing the Validity of a Self-Report Health Scale,* unpublished report, University of Louisville, Urban Studies Center, Louisville, Kentucky, 1984.

22. M. Stroebe and W. Stroebe, Who Suffers More? Sex Differences in Health Risks of the Widowed, *Psychological Bulletin, 93*, pp. 279-301, 1983.

23. P. Schulte and S. A. Murrell, *Kentucky Social Service Needs Assessment, The Telephone Survey*: Appendix B, University of Louisville, Urban Studies Center, Louisville, Kentucky, 1980.

24. S. A. Murrell, F. Norris, and G. L. Hutchins, Distribution and Desirability of Life Events in Older Adults: Population and Policy Implications, *Journal of Community Psychology, 12,* pp. 301-311, 1984.

25. S. A. Murrell, S. Himmelfarb, P. J. Schulte, and F. Norris, *Pretest of Candidate Measures: Results and Final Decisions,* Working Paper No. 9, Grant No. MH33063, University of Louisville, Urban Studies Center, Louisville, Kentucky, 1981.

Section III

Health Care System and Utilization Patterns

Chapter 12

RACE, GENDER, AND THE EFFECT OF SOCIAL SUPPORTS ON THE USE OF HEALTH SERVICES BY ELDERLY INDIVIDUALS

Martha A. Nelson

With the recognition of the heterogeneity of elderly individuals occurring in the past two decades [1], it is not surprising that many areas dealing with elderly persons remain under-researched. For example, among the studies dealing with the use of health services by elderly individuals, one area that has been largely ignored is the effects of social supports. Instead, many other factors have been treated as major determinants of this behavior.

Several studies [2] base their research on the behavioral model [3] that sees health services use as a function of the predisposing, enabling, and need characteristics of an individual. Studies using the behavioral model [2, 4-6] have been able to explain only low to moderate amounts of the variance in the use of health services. Additionally, most studies conclude that once the need factors are taken into account, the enabling and predisposing factors explain little variance in utilization [2, 6-8]. Because less than 30 percent of the variance in health services use has been explained by the behavioral model and because most studies fail to consider the role of social support, the present study looks at informal social supports as a potentially significant predictor of physician and hospital use among elderly individuals.

Social supports play a significant role in the lives of elderly individuals. Research on social support has shown that supportive relationships are associated with lower illness rates, faster recovery rates, and higher levels of health-care behavior [9]. People with few social contacts are less likely to use preventive health behaviors such as having health insurance or routine dental and medical checkups [10]. Elderly individuals prefer care from informal sources over formal sources [11] with kinship networks being the preferred source of social support

[12]. Currently, 70 percent of the disabled elderly living in the community with activity limitations receive all their care from spouses, relatives, or friends [13]. With the population of elderly individuals expected to increase to 17 percent of the U.S. total by the year 2020 [14], it is important to understand if the social support systems for elderly individuals act to increase or decrease their use of health services.

Few studies focus on social support as a major indicator of health services utilization, and their findings are contradictory. Krause found that social supports, as a whole, had limited additive effects on physician utilization [15]. Wan and Odell reported that the availability of social support was not a significant predictor of health services use [2]. In a subsequent study, however, Wan found that the availability of instrumental support and a social interaction network had a direct positive influence on the use of health services [16]. These discrepancies might be because social support is defined and measured differently across studies [17, 18]. The support process has been discussed in terms of the structure of an inter-personal relationship or network or in terms of the functions that a relationship or network serve [19]. Without a universal definition or measure of social support it is difficult to compare social support research.

Not only have the additive effects of social supports on the use of health services been neglected in the literature, so too has been the potential for inter-active effects. Social support systems differ by race and gender. Health services utilization also differs by race and gender. Accordingly, there is reason to believe that the effect of social supports on the use of health services by elderly indi-viduals may also differ by race and gender.

Numerous studies have examined how social support systems differ by race and gender. Many studies support the view that elderly African Americans have more pervasive social support networks than elderly white Americans. Specifically, elderly African-Americans interact and depend on kin in place of the non-familial institutions that provide support to white families [20]; church is an important coping and social support mechanism for African Americans [21, 22]; the effect of the informal support systems on reducing stress differs between African-Americans and whites [17, 23]; and African American families have been found to be more involved in exchanges of help across generations [24].

Many other studies suggest that significant differences have not been found between African Americans and whites with regard to informal supports and a few studies question the importance of ethnicity as a significant predictor of informal social supports. For example, elderly African Americans have not been found to have a greater potential for support from relatives [25], the social networks and support systems of elderly African Americans and whites have been found to be remarkably alike [23], and race may only affect social support indirectly through economic factors [17, 26]. Additionally, Rosenthal advises that gerontology should avoid assuming that ethnic families represent a traditional family type, with the connotation that they are, by definition, highly supportive of elderly individuals [27].

Unlike the literature on racial differences in social supports, studies on gender differences agree that differences do exist in the social networks and social worlds of men and women. Women have broader social ranges than men [28-31] and women turn to their intimate ties in times of need more so than men [28, 29]. Other similar findings suggest that women have larger social support networks [32, 33] and a greater number of close relationships than men [33]. Less certainty exists regarding whether women have more frequent social contact than men. For example, several studies report that women have more social contact than men [29, 32, 34] but another finds that men have more [28]. Additionally, Wright reports that differences in men's and women's friendships lessen as the strength and duration of friendships increase [35] and gender differences in social support are conditional on the events or circumstances that cause them to seek out support [36].

Racial and gender differences in the use of health services are reported frequently in the literature. Several studies report that some racial differences exist in the number of hospital or physician visits. These studies have reported that non-whites are least likely to be hospitalized [37, 38], a higher proportion of whites use mental health services [7], African Americans have a higher average number of physician visits, and white women are more likely to use private physicians than any other group [38]. One of the most consistent findings in the literature is that females are more likely than males to visit the doctor [39-43].

The literature reviewed in this section indicates that the studies using the behavioral model have only been able to explain about 30 percent of the variance in health services utilization, that these studies fail to consider social support as a major indicator, and that both social support systems and health service utilization differ by race and gender. Accordingly, the goal of this study is to examine two hypotheses. The first hypothesis examines the question: Does adding social support variables to the behavioral model increase the amount of variance explained? The second hypothesis examines an additional question: Do race and gender differences exist in the effect of social supports on the use of health services by elderly individuals?

METHODOLOGY

Data

This study utilizes secondary data that was originally compiled by the National Center for Health Statistics (NCHS). NCHS annually conducts the National Health Interview Survey (NHIS), interviewing a total of 42,000 households in the United States selected in a multistage probability sampling process. In 1984 the NHIS survey was extended to create the Longitudinal Study on Aging (LSOA). The LSOA consists of the 16,148 people aged fifty-five and over who were living in the 42,000 households included in the NHIS. The present study uses the subsample of the LSOA data consisting of 5,151 respondents aged seventy and over at the time of their 1984 interviews, who were followed for six years through multiple methods of data collection such as interviews and linkage with records. Fitti and Kovar offer detailed information regarding the design of the LSOA [44]. Because this study focuses on differences between whites and African-Americans, the fifty-six non-white, non-African American respondents were dropped from the analysis, resulting in an adjusted sample size of 5,095.

Measures

The conceptual framework to be used in this study will be the behavioral model developed by Andersen that includes predisposing, enabling, and need characteristics [3]. For this study, traditional measures of these characteristics have been selected [1]. The predisposing characteristics include age (a set of three dummy variables with the age group 70 to 74 as the reference category), gender, race, education (measured in number of years), and employment status. Enabling characteristics include income (measured in $1,000s), availability of insurance, having a telephone, and city size (a set of two dummy variables with small city as the reference category). Need characteristics include activities of daily living (ADL's), instrumental activities of daily living (IADL's), and perceived health status (respondents were asked to rate their health as excellent, very good, good, fair, or poor).

Health services were measured by contact and volume measures of physician visits and hospital visits. Contact measures are binary indicators of whether or not the respondent visited a physician or was admitted to the hospital in the past twelve months prior to the interview. Volume measures included the actual number of visits to a physician and the number of days spent in the hospital in the past twelve months, among those with contact. It was necessary to truncate the number of physician visits at thirteen and the number of days spent in the hospital at fifteen in order to correct for the positively skewed distributions [6, 8].

In studying the effects of social support on stress, Krause noted that when using an aggregate index of social support, it is impossible to evaluate whether all forms of social support buffer the impact of stress or if only certain types of supportive behavior buffer the impact of stress [45]. A subsequent study by Krause emphasizes this same message that aggregate indices of social support make it difficult to determine which form of supportive behavior (informational, instrumental, emotional, etc.) affects health behavior and health services use [15]. Following this advice, the present study uses eight measures of social support to better understand how different types of supportive behavior affect health services utilization.

The availability and frequency of contact with informal social supports were measured by dichotomous (yes/no) responses to questions regarding whether or not the respondent had any living siblings or children, spoke on the phone with relatives and friends in the past two weeks, got together with relatives and friends over the past two weeks, attended church or the temple in the past two weeks, and whether or not the respondent lived alone. The variable marital status indicates whether or not one is married, not whether or not one lives alone [46]; therefore, living alone has been chosen over marital status as a better indicator of the availability of social support.

Additionally, because this study uses secondary data, only the structural issues of social support are addressed. The focus of this study is on the availability of social networks as a potential resource to provide social support. Therefore, questions measuring the functional issues and quality of support, such as "what types of support are received from one's social network?" and "are they satisfactory?" cannot be explored. Table 1 provides a list of the coding algorithms, means, standard deviations, and number of respondents for all the variables.

Design

For this study, the use of health services will be seen as a function of the predisposing, enabling, and need characteristics, and of informal social supports. To test how well the informal social support variables predict health services, a two-stage model is needed. In the first stage, health services use will be regressed on the predisposing, enabling, and need characteristics. In the second stage, health services use will be regressed on the predisposing, enabling, and need characteristics plus the informal social support measures. By comparing the explained variance of these two regression equations with F Ratios, we will be able to see if the unique additive effects of informal supports offer any further explanation in predicting health services use. The additive effects will be indexed by the partial regression coefficients of the social support measures.

The second purpose of this study is to explore the differences in the effects informal social supports have on the use of health services among elderly African Americans and white males and females. In doing this it is necessary to partition the data. The regression equation, then, will be estimated separately within each race and gender group (i.e., among African American males, African American females, white males, and white females). The resulting unstandardized, partial regression coefficients will be compared across groups by constructing confidence intervals around each parameter estimate. If the coefficients pertaining to each subpopulation fall within the 95 percent confidence interval of the remaining subpopulations and vice versa, then the effect of informal social supports on health services use is consistent across the four race and gender groups. If the

Table 1. Coding Algorithms, Number of Respondents, Means, and Standard Deviations of All Variables (*N* = 5095)

Variable	Coding Algorithm	N	Mean	Standard Deviation
Predisposing Characteristics				
Age Group 2 (75-79)	1 = Yes 0 = No	1309 3786	.257	.437
Age Group 3 (80-84)	1 = Yes 0 = No	1248 3847	.245	.430
Age Group 4 (85-89)	1 = Yes 0 = No	820 4275	.161	.368
Education	Number of Years	4997	9.777	3.720
Female	1 = Yes 0 = No	3265 1830	.641	.480
Employment	1 = Yes 0 = No	429 4666	.084	.278
African American	1 = Yes 0 = No	560 4535	.110	.313
Enabling Characteristics				
Big City	1 = Yes 0 = No	1713 3382	.336	.472
Non-City	1 = Yes 0 = No	1944 3151	.382	.486
Health Insurance	1 = Yes 0 = No	3448 1647	.677	.468
Income	$1,000's	5095	13.210	10.590
Phone	1 = Yes 0 = No	4936 159	.969	.174
Need Characteristics				
Perceived Health Status	1 = Excellent, Very Good, or Good 0 = Fair, or Poor	3362 1733	.660	.474
Activities of Daily Living	Number of ADL's with need for help	5063	.792	1.584

Table 1. (Cont'd.)

Variable	Coding Algorithm	N	Mean	Standard Deviation
Instrumental Activities of Daily Living	Number of IADL's with need for help	5059	.827	1.502
Social Support Variables				
Living Children	1 = Yes 0 = No	4293 802	.843	.364
Living Siblings	2 = Brothers and Sisters 0 = No Siblings	3807 1288	1.107	.775
Get Together With Friends in Past 2 Weeks	1 = Yes 0 = No	3447 1648	.677	.468
Get Together With Relatives in Past 2 Weeks	1 = Yes 0 = No	3916 1179	.769	.422
Talk on Phone With Friends in Past 2 Weeks	1 = Yes 0 = No	3978 1117	.781	.414
Talk on Phone With Relatives in Past 2 Weeks	1 = Yes 0 = No	4263 832	.837	.370
Go to Church, Temple Past 2 Weeks	1 = Yes 0 = No	2522 2573	.495	.500
Live Alone	1 = Yes 0 = No	1902 3193	.373	.484
Measures of Health Services Utilization				
Seen a Physician in Past Year	1 = Yes 0 = No	4238 857	.832	.374
Number of Physician Visits (of those with physician contact; visits truncated at 13)	Actual Number	4238	5.160	4.022
Stayed in Hospital Overnight in Past Year	1 = Yes 0 = No	1115 3980	.219	.414
Number of Days Spent in the Hospital (of those with hospital contact; days truncated at 15)	Actual Number	1115	8.846	4.989

coefficients for each subpopulation do not fall within the 95 percent confidence intervals, then the effect of informal supports on physician and hospital utilization by elderly individuals is specified by race and gender.

RESULTS

Additive Effects

Table 2 presents the results of testing the first stage model, in which social supports are excluded. For simplicity, only those effects significant at or beyond the .05 level are shown. Table 2 illustrates that the more predisposed one is, the more enabled one is, and the more need one has, the greater the use of health services. The need characteristics show generally consistent significant effects across all measures of health services use and are the most powerful predictors. Perceiving one's health as fair or poor and having ADL's or IADL's significantly affect health services use.

Table 2 also shows that the factors in the behavioral model account for low amounts of variance in all the dependent variables. The model explains 3.24 percent of the variance in physician contact, 12.72 percent in the number of physician visits, 7.46 percent in hospital contact, and 5.58 percent in the number of days spent in the hospital. These figures are in the range of the results found in the literature.

It was hypothesized that adding social support variables to the behavioral model would increase the variance explained by the model. Table 3 provides support for this hypothesis and shows an increase in the amount of variance explained in health services utilization when the social support variables are added into the model (after the predisposing, enabling, and need characteristics). The R^2s increase to 3.71 percent for physician contact, 13.2 percent for the number of physician visits, 7.59 percent for hospital contact, and 6.8 percent for the number of days spent in the hospital. Although the R^2 increments are minimal, performing F tests on the increments indicate that social supports have statistically significant unique additive effects on both measures of physician utilization and the number of days spent in the hospital. This statistical significance, however, likely results more from the large sample size than from the magnitude of the effect. Nevertheless, the results support the first research hypothesis that adding social support variables to the behavioral model further explains the use of health services. Additionally, a few of the social support indicators had statistically significant effects.

Whether or not one attended church had a more consistent effect across the dependent variables than any of the other social support indicators. For all the dependent variables, except physician contact, those respondents indicating that they did not attend church or temple in the two weeks prior to the interview were more likely to have more physician visits and hospital contact and

Table 2. Unstandardized Partial Regression and R^2 Coefficients of the Predisposing, Enabling, and Need Characteristics on Physician and Hospital Utilization Measures

| | Physician Visits | | Hospital Visits | |
| | Contact $N = 4962$ | Volume $N = 4140$ | Contact $N = 4962$ | Volume $N = 1083$ |
Independent Variable				
Predisposing Characteristics				
Age Group 2			.033[a]	
Age Group 3	.033[a]			
Age Group 4		−.467[a]		
Female			−.030[a]	−.827[b]
African American			−.066[c]	1.204[a]
Education				
Employment		−.649[b]		
Enabling Characteristics				
Income	.013[a]	.117[a]	.016[b]	
Insurance	.072[c]			
Big City		.349[a]		
Non-City	−.036[b]			
Phone	.106		.071[a]	
Need Characteristics				
IADL	.015[b]	.183[b]	.028[c]	.270[a]
ADL		.263[c]	.022[c]	.282[b]
Perceived Health	−.080[c]	−2.112[c]	−.140[c]	−.875[b]
Intercept	.697	5.269	.194	7.362
R^2	.0324[c]	.1272[c]	.0746[c]	.0558[c]

[a]Significant at .05
[b]Significant at .01
[c]Significant at .001

a higher number of days spent in the hospital than those who attended church or temple. For physician contact, however, those who did not attend church or temple were less likely to have contacted a physician in the past year than those who did attend.

Interactive Effects

To determine whether or not racial and gender differences existed in the effects of social supports on health services use, both significant and insignificant unstandardized regression coefficients were compared. Because of a limited number of

Table 3. Unstandardized Partial Regression and R^2 Coefficients
of the Social Support Variables on Physician and
Hospital Utilization Measures

	Physician Visits		Hospital Visits	
Independent Variable	Contact $N = 4962$	Volume $N = 4140$	Contact $N = 4962$	Volume $N = 1083$
Social Support Variables				
Talk on the Phone With Relatives	.035[a]			
Talk on the Phone With Friends		.439[a]		−1.012[a]
Get Together With Relatives				
Get Together With Friends				
Presence of Living Children				
Presence of Living Siblings				
Live Alone		.370[b]		
Church Attendance	.028[a]	−.42[c]	−.03[a]	−.746[a]
Intercept	.643	5.297	.209	8.024
R^2 (without support variables)[d]	.0324	.1272	.0746	.0558
R^2 (with support variables)[d]	.0371[c]	.132[c]	.0759	.068[a]

[a]Significant at .05
[b]Significant at .01
[c]Significant at .001
[d]R^2s include predisposing, enabling, and need variables

cases, no comparisons of how social supports affected the number of days spent in the hospital between African American males and the three remaining groups were made. Following Wolinsky, statistically significant racial and gender differences exist when the regression coefficient for a given independent variable on a particular dependent variable in one subpopulation falls outside of the 95 percent confidence interval of the regression coefficient for the same independent variable in another subpopulation and vice versa [8].

It was hypothesized that race and gender differences exist in the effect of social supports on elderly individual's use of health services. Table 4 provides support for this hypothesis and indicates that several racial and gender differences existed in the effects of five of the eight support variables on physician contact, however no consistent patterns emerged. Talking on the phone with friends positively affected physician contact for all the groups except African American females. African American females were more likely to contact a physician when they did not talk on the phone with friends and this was a statistically significant effect.

The effects of getting together with relatives on physician contact differed between African American males and females. African American males who got together with their relatives contacted a physician more, but when they got together with their friends physician contact decreased. The inverse was true for African American females. When they got together with their relatives physician contact decreased but increased when they got together with their friends and this effect was statistically significant. Furthermore, the effect that getting together with friends had on physician contact differed between African American and white females. The effect was positive for African American females and negative for white females.

The presence of siblings had a statistically significant effect on physician contact for white males. White males with siblings were less likely to contact a physician. The opposite was true for both groups of females. They were more likely to visit a physician when siblings existed.

Living alone was the final support variable to differentially affect physician contact. African American females were significantly more likely to contact a physician when living alone than were white males and females. Differences also existed between white males and females. White females who lived with others contacted a physician more than white males who lived with others.

Table 5 indicates that only three of the eight social support variables showed a racial and/or gender difference in their effect on the number of physician visits. The only social support variable to show a racial and gender difference was church attendance, and it had a negative effect on the number of physician visits for all groups except African American females. The effect of this variable was statistically significant for both white females and African American males and strongest for African American males. African American males were much more likely to have visited a physician when they did not attend church.

Two other support variables differed, by gender, in their effect on the number of physician visits. The first support variable, talking on the phone with friends, had a positive effect for both white males and females, but the effect was stronger and statistically significant for the males. The second support variable, getting together with relatives, had a negative effect on the number of physician visits for African-American males and a positive effect for African American females.

Table 4. Unstandardized Partial Regression Coefficients and Standard Errors (in Parentheses) of the Social Support Variables on Physician Contact

Social Support Variable	Physician Contact				Significant Differences in Effect of Social Support Variables
	White Males N = 1599	African American Males N = 188	White Females N = 2825	African American Females N = 347	
Talk on the Phone With Relatives	.041 (.029)	.076 (.091)	.016 (.024)	.049 (.064)	
Talk on the Phone With Friends	.024 (.025)	.066 (.08)	.017 (.022)	$-.143^a$ (.066)	African American Females different from all
Get Together With Relatives	.026 (.025)	.15 (.086)	.019 (.018)	$-.05$ (.045)	African American Males different from African American Females
Get Together With Friends	.028 (.022)	$-.021$ (.068)	$-.003$ (.017)	$.091^a$ (.042)	African American Females different from African American Males and White Females
Presence of Living Children	.017 (.025)	$-.064$ (.079)	.029 (.017)	$-.004$ (.041)	
Presence of Living Siblings	$-.03^a$ (.013)	.041 (.042)	.005 (.009)	.044 (.026)	White Males different from African American and White Females
Live Alone	$-.039$ (.026)	.023 (.088)	.024 (.015)	$.122^b$ (.042)	African American Females different from White Males and Females
Church Attendance	.028 (.02)	$-.024$ (.074)	.026 (.015)	.069 (.044)	
R^2 (without support variables)[d]	.0324				
R^2 (with support variables)[d]	$.0371^c$				

[a] Significant at .05
[b] Significant at .01
[c] Significant at .001
[d] R^2's include all predisposing, enabling, and need variables

Table 5. Unstandardized Partial Regression Coefficients and Standard Errors (in Parentheses) of the Social Support Variables on the Number of Physician Visits of Those Who Contacted a Physician

Social Support Variable	Number of Physician Visits				Significant Differences in Effect of Social Support Variables
	White Males $N = 1316$	African American Males $N = 145$	White Females $N = 2380$	African American Females $N = 296$	
Talk on the Phone With Relatives	.158 (.324)	.504 (1.028)	.18 (28)	.013 (.811)	
Talk on the Phone With Friends	.738[b] (.28)	1.153 (.917)	.114 (.247)	1.151 (.806)	White Males different from White Females
Get Together With Relatives	−.151 (.277)	−1.397 (1.001)	.005 (.209)	.887 (.57)	African American Males different from African American Females
Get Together With Friends	−.43 (.246)	.992 (.797)	−.096 (.189)	−.335 (.528)	
Presence of Living Children	−.188 (.278)	−.049 (.883)	−.012 (.198)	−.734 (.515)	
Presence of Living Siblings	.017 (.142)	−.027 (.477)	.013 (.105)	.169 (.326)	
Live Alone	.554 (.289)	.73 (1.01)	.201 (.175)	.445 (.536)	
Church Attendance	−.339 (.22)	−2.211[a] (.872)	−.415[a] (.166)	.183 (.559)	African American Females different from all
R^2 (without support variables)[d]	.1272				
R^2 (with support variables)[d]	.1320[c]				

[a] Significant at .05
[b] Significant at .01
[c] Significant at .001
[d] R^2's include all predisposing, enabling, and need variables

193

Racial and gender differences were not found in the effects of the social support variables on hospital contact and only one support variable, getting together with relatives, had an effect on the number of days spent in the hospital.[1] Considering that hospital admissions are primarily made according to the degree of illness [47] rather than on socioeconomic criteria, this finding is not unexpected. Two social support variables, talking on the phone with relatives and the presence of living children, showed absolutely no racial and gender differences in their effect on any physician or hospital utilization measure.

DISCUSSION AND CONCLUSION

This study has attempted to provide further insight into the study of elderly adult's health behavior. Specifically, the focus has been on analyzing the effects that social supports have on certain physician and hospital utilization measures. The results reported in this study confirm both research hypotheses that social supports have additive and interactive effects on elderly individual's use of health services. It is important to keep in mind that this study was not able to uncover the specific reasons underlying the role of social supports in elderly individual's use of physicians and hospitals, therefore, this discussion is based partly on speculation. For clarification purposes, only the most salient additive and interactive effects are discussed.

Additive Effects

Although adding the support variables to the behavioral model increased the R^2s only minimally, the increments for both measures of physician use and the number of days spent in the hospital were statistically significant. Inclusion of both structural and functional measures of support may have resulted in substantial increments in the R^2s. The only support variable to have consistent, statistically significant effects across all four dependent variables was church attendance.

Church attendance was found to have a consistent significant effect across both physician and hospitalization measures. One interpretation suggests that there is something about attending church, whether it be the religion itself, or the church community, that appears to encourage or influence one to visit the doctor for an annual check-up to prevent illnesses or to seek treatment for some existing health problem. Literature dealing with religious commitment and health notes that religious commitment has been viewed as a type of

---

[1] Because race and gender differences were not found in the effects of the social support variables on hospital contact and only one social support variable had an effect on the number of days spent in the hospital, these two tables were excluded.

social support that encourages preventive health practices such as visits to physicians [10, 48].

Furthermore, if the church or its community encourages physician contact as a preventive health measure, then this might reduce the need for future health services use, and help explain why church has a significantly negative effect on the number of physician visits and the two measures of hospital utilization. This interpretation is in line with several studies [10, 49] reporting that those who attend church frequently have lower illness rates. Lower illness rates, in turn, decrease some of the need for physician and hospital use. The fact that church attendance significantly affected all measures of physician and hospital utilization supports the current literature [9, 10, 48, 49] that church attendance is a very important factor in predicting health services use.

Given the fact that much of the social support literature speaks of the importance of siblings and children as the preferred health care providers, it is surprising that these two variables were insignificant. It is possible that these two variables might have shown significant effects on the use of health services if functional measures, in addition to structural measures, would have been available for analysis. These functional measures might have consisted of asking the respondent if children and siblings were sources of support and what type of support was received from them.

Interactive Effects

One's understanding of elderly adult's health behavior is further enriched by reviewing the racial and gender differences that were found in the effects of social supports on physician and hospital use. First of all, no racial and gender differences were found in the effects of talking on the phone with relatives, or the presence of living children. As well, no racial and gender differences were found in the effects of any of the social support variables on hospital contact. This finding is not surprising when one considers the fact that hospital admissions are predominantly the result of non-discretionary behavior [47].

Although several racial and gender differences were found in the effects of the support variables on the other measures of health services, it is difficult to make general conclusions. The effect of a social support variable within the same racial and gender group did not have the same effect across each measure of health services use. For example, African American females were more likely to have contacted a physician and spent more days in the hospital when they did not get together with relatives. Yet, they reported more physician visits when they did get together with relatives. The opposite was true for African American males. One interpretation suggests that getting together with relatives substituted for the need of African American females to contact a physician, whereas, for African American males, it encouraged physician contact. If the relatives act as a substitute for physician contact this may cause the health condition to worsen until a number of visits are inevitable. African American males who might have been encouraged by relatives to visit the physician upon first acknowledging a health concern, may have cleared up the health problem in its beginning stages and eliminated the need for subsequent physician visits.

One of the most consistent findings in this study was that gender differences existed in the effects of the support variables on physician and hospital use. For example, white males were more likely to visit the physician in the absence of siblings than were white and African American females, and this support variable was statistically significant for white males. This finding suggests that the presence of siblings, as a provider of social support, substitutes for the need for white males to contact a physician, while for African American and white females, the presence of siblings encourages them to contact a physician as other studies have indicated [2, 16].

The effect of living alone on physician contact also differed by gender. White males who live alone are less likely to visit a physician but white and African American females who live alone are more likely to visit a physician. This finding supports the idea that white males depend upon those they live with to encourage and persuade them to contact a physician [10].

A gender difference was also found in the effect of talking on the phone with friends on the number of physician visits. Although for both white males and females the number of physician visits increased with talking on the phone with friends, the effect was statistically significant for white males. One interpretation is concerned with the fact that males and females suffer from different disorders [17] that require different types and amounts of formal health care. Although the nature of the phone conversations and the reasons for visiting the doctor are unknown, for the females, talking on the phone with friends about their health problems might have been a sufficient substitute for professional help or it might have acted to prevent the onset of future health problems. For the males, their friends might have encouraged them to visit a doctor.

Although the relatively small sample size for the African American males and females creates a bit of skepticism in these results, it is possible to conclude that friends and relatives serve different functions for males and females with regard to physician and hospital utilization. It appears that whether friends or relatives act to encourage, substitute for, or prevent the use of health services depends upon the illness or health concern at hand. These results support the views that the social worlds of men and women differ greatly [28-30] and that how social support systems differ by gender are conditional on the events or circumstances that cause males and females to seek support [36].

The final major finding from analyzing the interactive effects of race and gender on health services utilization was that church attendance was found to have significant interactive effects. African American males who did not attend church were five times more likely to have numerous physician visits than any other group, especially African American females whose number of physician visits was positively affected by attending church. Following the findings of Berkman and Syme, who report that church membership encourages the use of preventive health behaviors such as medical check-ups [10], one would expect that African American males, as well as white males and females, who attend church would have more physician visits. Instead, the results suggest that, for African American males, a high number of physician visits occurred even though church attendance was very low. In contrast, the effect of church attendance for African American females on the number of physician visits was positive, indicating that attending church may have encouraged more physician use. Knowing the type of support that was received by attending church and the medical reasons for the physician visit would help explain these findings.

This study contributes to the research on elderly individuals use of health services in at least three ways. First, the results indicate that a modestly significant relationship exists between social supports, especially the effect of church, and the use of health services among the elderly individuals. The inclusion of a functional measure of support in the behavioral model that reveals how religion, church attendance, membership or some other measure of religiosity serves as a source of support for elderly individuals and the type of support received from this source might help to further increase the explained variance. Second, this study supports the current literature that the social worlds of men and women differ greatly. Finally, this study reports that the effect of social supports on the use of health services by elderly individuals differs by race and gender. However, these differences were not consistent across the various measures of health services utilization supporting the finding in the literature that elderly individuals are a diverse group.

Overall, this study suggests that the relationship between social supports and health services use is complex. If the substitution of informal supports for formal care is one way to keep the formal support system from becoming overwhelmed in the future, it is imperative to understand thoroughly what type of support is received from which sources, how supports encourage the use of formal care, and how social supports substitute for and prevent the need for formal care within all race and gender groups.

REFERENCES

1. F. D. Wolinsky and C. Arnold, A Different Perspective on Health and Health Services Utilization, *Annual Review of Gerontology and Geriatrics, 8*, pp. 7-101, 1988.
2. T. H. Wan and B. G. Odell, Factors Affecting the Use of Social and Health Services Among the Elderly, *Aging and Society, 1*(March), pp. 95-115, 1981.
3. R. Andersen, *A Behavioral Model of Families' Use of Health Services,* Center for Health Administration Studies, Chicago, 1968.

4. C. Evashwick et al., Factors Explaining the Use of Health Care Services by the Elderly, *Health Services Research, 19*:3, pp. 357-382, 1984.
5. L. Branch et al., Toward Understanding Elders' Health Service Utilization, *Journal of Community Health, 7*:2, pp. 80-91, 1981.
6. F. D. Wolinsky and R. M. Coe, Physician and Hospital Utilization Among Noninstitutionalized Elderly Adults: An Analysis of the Health Interview Survey, *Journal of Gerontology, 39*:3, pp. 334-341, 1984.
7. C. Coulton and A. K. Frost, Use of Social and Health Services by the Elderly, *Journal of Health and Social Behavior, 23*:December, pp. 330-339, 1982.
8. F. D. Wolinsky et al., Ethnic Differences in the Demand for Physician and Hospital Utilization Among Older Adults in Major American Cities, *The Milbank Quarterly, 67*, pp. 412-449, 1989.
9. W. A. McIntosh and P. A. Shifflett, Influence of Social Support Systems on Dietary Intake of the Elderly, *Journal of Nutrition for the Elderly, 4*:1, pp. 5-18, 1984.
10. L. F. Berkman and S. L. Syme, Social Networks, Host Resistance, and Mortality: A Nine-Year Follow-up Study of Alameda County Residents, *American Journal of Epidemiology, 109*:2, pp. 186-204, 1979.
11. M. Cantor and V. Little, Aging and Social Care, in *Handbook of Aging and the Social Sciences,* R. Binstock and E. Shanas (eds.), Reinhold, New York, 1985.
12. M. Cantor, Neighbors and Friends: An Overlooked Resource in the Informal Support System, *Research on Aging, 1*:4, pp. 434-463, 1979.
13. U.S. Department of Health and Human Services, Personnel for Health Needs of the Elderly Through the Year 2020, in *Report to Congress,* National Institute on Aging, Maryland, 1987.
14. U.S. Bureau of the Census, Projections of the Population of the United States, by Age, Sex, and Race: 1988-2080, in *Current Population Reports,* Series P-25, No. 1018, U.S. Government Printing Office, Washington, D.C., 1989.
15. N. Krause, Stressful Life Events and Physician Utilization, *Journal of Gerontology, 43*:2, pp. S53-S61, 1988.
16. T. H. Wan, Functionally Disabled Elderly, *Research on Aging, 9*:1, pp. 61-78, 1987.
17. N. Krause, Gender and Ethnicity Differences in Psychological Well-Being, *Annual Review of Gerontology and Geriatrics, 8,* pp. 156-188, 1988.
18. N. Krause, The Measurement of Social Support in Studies on Aging and Health, in *Aging, Stress, Social Support, and Health,* K. Markides and C. Cooper (eds.), Wiley and Sons, New York, 1989.
19. S. Cohen and S. L. Syme, Issues in the Study of and Application of Social Support, *Social Support and Health,* Academic Press, Orlando, 1985.
20. W. C. Hays and C. H. Mindel, Extended Kinship Relations in Black and White Families, *Journal of Marriage and the Family,* pp. 51-56, February 1973.
21. K. Conway, Coping With the Stress of Medical Problems Among Black and White Elderly, *International Journal of Aging and Human Development, 21*:1, pp. 39-47, 1985.
22. L. R. Hatch, Informal Support Patterns of Older African-American and White Women, *Research on Aging, 13*:2, pp. 144-170, 1991.
23. D. E. Biegel et al., Social Support Networks of White and Black Elderly People at Risk for Institutionalization, *Health and Social Work, 16*:4, pp. 245-257, 1991.

24. E. Mutran, Intergenerational Family Support Among Blacks and Whites: Response to Culture or to SES Differences, *Journal of Gerontology, 40*:3, pp. 382-389, 1985.

25. M. Cantor, The Informal Support System of New York's Inner City Elderly: Is Ethnicity a Factor?, in *Ethnicity and Aging,* D. E. Gelfand and A. J. Kutzik (eds.), Springer, New York, 1979.

26. C. H. Mindel et al., Informal and Formal Health and Social Support Systems of Black and White Elderly: A Comparative Cost Approach, *The Gerontologist, 26*:3, pp. 279-285, 1986.

27. C. Rosenthal, Family Supports in Later Life: Does Ethnicity Make a Difference?, *The Gerontologist, 26*:1, pp. 19-24, 1986.

28. E. A. Powers and G. L. Bultena, Sex Differences in Intimate Friendships of Old Age, *Journal of Marriage and the Family,* pp. 740-747, November 1976.

29. T. C. Antonucci, Personal Characteristics, Social Support and Social Behavior, in *Handbook of Aging and the Social Sciences,* R. Binstock and E. Shanas (eds.), Reinhold, New York, 1985.

30. R. L. Kahn and T. C. Antonucci, *Social Supports of the Elderly: Family, Friends, Professionals,* in Final Report to the National Institute on Aging, 1983.

31. J. Kohen, Old But Not Alone: Informal Social Supports Among the Elderly by Marital Status and Sex, *The Gerontologist, 23*:1, pp. 57-63, 1983.

32. G. Arling, Strain, Social Support and Distress in Old Age, *Journal of Gerontology, 42,* pp. 107-113, 1987.

33. C. Depner and B. Ingersoll, Employment Status and Social Support: The Experience of the Mature Woman, in *Women's Retirement: Policy Implications for Recent Research,* M. Szinovacz (ed.), Sage, Beverly Hills, 1982.

34. L. M. Chatters et al., Size and Composition of the Informal Helper Networks of Elderly Blacks, *Journal of Gerontology, 40*:5, pp. 605-614, 1985.

35. P. Wright, Men's Friendships, Women's Friendships and the Alleged Inferiority of the Latter, *Sex Roles, 8*:1, pp. 1-20, 1982.

36. N. Krause and V. Keith, Gender Differences in Social Support among Older Adults, *Sex Roles, 21*:9, pp. 609-628, 1989.

37. E. Mutran and K. Ferraro, Medical Need and Use of Services among Older Men and Women, *Journal of Gerontology, 43*:5, pp. S162-171, 1988.

38. T. H. Wan, Use of Health Services by the Elderly in Low-Income Communities, *Milbank Memorial Fund Quarterly/Health and Society, 60*:1, pp. 82-107, 1982.

39. E. Stoller, Patterns of Physician Utilization by the Elderly: A Multivariate Analysis, *Medical Care, 20*:11, pp. 1080-1089, 1982.

40. N. P. Roos and E. Shapiro, The Manitoba Longitudinal Study on Aging: Preliminary Findings on Health Care Utilization by the Elderly, *Medical Care, 19*:6, pp. 644-657, 1981.

41. A. C. Marcus and J. M. Siegel, Sex Differences in the Use of Physician Services: A Preliminary Test of the Fixed Role Hypothesis, *Journal of Health and Social Behavior, 23*:September, pp. 186-197, 1982.

42. F. D. Wolinsky, Assessing the Effects of Predisposing, Enabling, and Illness-Morbidity Characteristics on Health Service Utilization, *Journal of Health and Social Behavior, 19*: pp. 384-396, December 1978.

43. P. D. Cleary et al., Sex Differences in Medical Care Utilization: An Empirical Investigation, *Journal of Health and Social Behavior, 23*, pp. 106-119, June 1982.
44. J. E. Fitti and M. G. Kovar, The Supplement on Aging to the 1984 National Health Interview Survey, *Vital Health and Statistics, 1*:21, 1987.
45. N. Krause, Social Support, Stress, and Well-Being among Older Adults, *Journal of Gerontology, 41*:4, pp. 512-519, 1986.
46. G. L. Cafferata, Marital Status, Living Arrangements, and the Use of Health Services by Elderly Persons, *Journal of Gerontology, 42*:6, pp. 613-618, 1987.
47. R. Andersen et al., *Equity in Health Services,* Ballinger, Cambridge, 1975.
48. J. K. Langlie, Social Networks, Health Beliefs, and Preventive Health Behavior, *Journal of Health and Social Behavior, 18*, pp. 244-260, September 1977.
49. G. W. Comstock and K. B. Partridge, Church Attendance and Health, *Journal of Chronic Diseases, 25,* pp. 665-672, 1972.

Chapter 13

IMPLICATIONS OF A MENTAL HEALTH INTERVENTION FOR ELDERLY MENTALLY ILL RESIDENTS OF RESIDENTIAL CARE FACILITIES

Leonard E. Gottesman
Ellen Peskin
Kathleen Kennedy
and
Jana Mossey

Demographic shifts toward the aging of the population, legislative changes that restrict admissions to nursing homes, and policy changes mandating the deinstitutionalization of the mentally ill have resulted in a dramatic increase in the number of mentally ill elderly persons who are receiving shelter and care in residential care facilities (boarding homes). In the United States, during 1987, there were 563,000 beds in 41,000 licensed facilities and an unknown but presumably large number of smaller unlicensed boarding homes [1].

Residential care facilities (RCFs) provide room and board and a variety of supportive services short of medical and nursing care. The mentally frail compose a major portion of their population. For example, the Denver Research Institute's national study [2] reported that 28 percent of residents in RCFs serving elderly people, and 77.9 percent of residents in RCFs serving the mentally ill, had previously lived in a psychiatric institution. Pennsylvania estimates that from 20 percent [3] to over 30 percent [4] of RCF residents have some mental illness diagnosis, and that the proportion of residents who are mentally ill increases directly with age [4].

There is evidence that the mentally ill in RCFs receive few mental health and medical services. Dittmar, et al. [2] report that over one-half of the elderly residents and one-third of the mentally ill residents in RCFs who needed mental health services did not receive them during a one-year period. Partial hospitalization or day program participation was observed for only 10 percent of the residents [5]. Similarly, Sherwood and Gruenberg reported that 99 percent of the elderly residents they studied needed physician services and/or hospital care, regardless of their mental health status [6]. There have been reports of inadequate review of prescriptions, unmet needs in the areas of hearing, dental care and eye exams, and nutritionally inadequate meals [5].

Few states require individualized care plans for the elderly or mentally ill residents within RCFs [7,8]. Operators, therefore, provide only those maintenance services their staffs and budgets allow. For example, the Denver study reported that 20 percent of the residents in RCFs for the mentally ill and older adults did not participate in any social activities within the facility [2]. Similarly, Faulk found that, other than the occasional celebration of a resident's birthday, 90 percent of homes did not provide any regular stimulative activities [5].

Service gaps to RCF residents may result from the providers' lack of familiarity with the resources available to their clients. It may also reflect the frustration and difficulty providers report encountering when attempting to navigate the professional service network in the community. Finally, residents may not receive services because of agency priorities. Many agencies that serve the mentally ill do not give priority to serving elderly persons, while agencies serving elderly persons often have little interest in serving the mentally ill. Since many RCF residents are both mentally ill and elderly, they may fall outside both service systems' priorities.

Another difficulty behind the limited services to the elderly mentally ill RCF resident may be characteristics of the residents themselves. Many residents have trouble managing travel, paying for it, or meeting the eligibility and scheduling requirements of special transportation. Furthermore, chronic and elderly ex-mental hospital patients generally have histories replete with failures, both rehabilitative and personal. These histories sometimes contribute to their reluctance to participate in those programs that are offered to them. Likewise, in developing this study, we found the prevailing notion among mental health professionals to be that aged RCF residents are the "lost causes" who have the least likelihood for long-term improvement.

POSSIBLE PROGRAMMATIC SOLUTIONS

Programs that may be successful in addressing the problems of RCF residents are described in studies of both institutional and community treatment of the mentally ill. For example, in the 1960's, prior to the first large scale release of long-term elderly mental hospital patients to the community, Donahue, Coons, and Gottesman developed and tested milieu treatment within a large mental hospital [9]. That project reported improved instrumental skills in both schizophrenic and organically impaired residents but only as long as program supports continued. Similarly, major programs of community care have demonstrated success with young ex-mental hospital patients when they were given opportunities for engaging in normal activities "in situ" [10,11]. Despite this success, however, these community programs have not typically addressed the particular needs of the older ex-mental hospital patient.

More recently, the Community Care Program was designed to compare community based foster care settings with nursing homes regarding the quality and costs of care provided for elderly persons with no viable family supports [12]. Offering the combined efforts of nursing, medical, and social service professionals, the program's goals were to prevent inappropriate institutionalization, minimize utilization of acute care, and provide a living environment that satisfies the clients' social, emotional, and physical needs. Evaluation of the program found that residents in foster care did better on functional measures, nursing goals, discharge, and mortality, while nursing home patients did better of life satisfaction, perceived health, and social recreation activities [13]. The investigators concluded that despite expenses for health and social services provided in foster care, the total cost of the community-based program was well below that for nursing home care [13, 14] but was still relatively high compared to typical RCF care.

Based on the apparent mental health needs of RCF residents of all ages, the Pennsylvania Office of Mental Health earmarked approximately $750,000 to county mental health authorities to provide mental health services to residents of licensed personal care homes. Partly because this commitment to enhancing mental health services in this locale was relatively rare, The National Institute of Mental Health (NIMH) awarded the authors a three year grant to evaluate the impact of these new services on elderly residents.

The original state guidelines for the intervention established few limits other than the requirement that the funds be used for personnel costs. The program was widely promoted and supported publicly by the Secretary of Welfare. There were few takers. County officials, generally, expressed concern that the funds were insufficient, and that the absence of a guarantee of continued funds in subsequent years might obligate them to provide more long-term support with local funds.

Delaware County, adjacent to Philadelphia, was one of only two counties that actually initiated a program. It divided the funds between a hospital-based community mental health center and a psychosocial rehabilitation program to provide personal care facilities in the County with additional mental health services.

With NIMH permission, the grant, designed originally to evaluate the statewide effort, was refocused to measure impact of the augmented mental health care in Delaware County. To support the emphasis on elderly residents, research funds were used to employ two additional half-time workers who concentrated on delivering services to mentally ill residents over the age of fifty.

This study measured the treatment impact by including a comparison group receiving "regular," mental health care in other facilities in another county. The specific hypotheses were that the intervention would 1) increase the amount of physical and mental health services received by experimental group residents, and 2) decrease the manifestation of physical and mental illness symptoms.

METHODS

The Intervention Program

The intervention had four components: 1) case management to increase the fit between residents' unattended problems and available but unused community resources; 2) psychosocial rehabilitation to engage residents assumed to be under-stimulated in normal instrumental and social behaviors; 3) individual counseling; and 4) training RCF staff to help them to better meet the resident needs and to increase their demands on their clients for more normal (i.e., non-institutional) behavior.

The intervention involved four workers. Two half-time workers were on the research project payroll, one full-time worker was employed by the mental health center, while the fourth worked full time for the psychosocial rehabilitation center. A full-time caseload was forty residents. Although the residents did receive all components of the intervention, the workers designed individualized interventions that met the particular needs of the resident and that were compatible with whatever services they were already receiving.

A great deal of the two full-time workers' programmatic efforts were similar in focus although each was constrained by the priorities of her parent agency. Both the mental health center worker and the psychosocial program worker met regularly with small groups of residents for discussions aimed at life skills development. These discussions concerned such topics as appropriate dress, engaging in social interactions effectively, following medication regimes, proper management of drinking, and so on. The psychosocial rehabilitation center also involved some residents in programs at an off-site program. Other residents who attended a private mental health center three times weekly participated in similar group and individual activities. The interventions designed by the four workers included one on one socialization, arranging for glasses, dentures and other medically related matters, and getting the residents included in programs at the local senior center.

The Study Sample

All thirteen licensed personal care homes in Delaware County were invited to participate in the study. The six facilities that agreed to cooperate included two that were already receiving augmented services and four others. All six predominately served residents receiving Social Security Insurance (SSI) or having a history of mental illness.

Facilities within two areas of Philadelphia were targeted by the comparison group. Fourteen of twenty-eight homes with a capacity for at least ten residents agreed to participate. All these homes: 1) had at least four residents with an apparent need for mental health services; 2) served an elderly population; and 3) were not affiliated with and did not share premises with a mental health center.

The resident capacity of the combined sample of twenty experimental and comparison RCFs was 1,007, and a convenience sample was drawn from among the 279 residents providers identified as: 1) at least 50 years of age; and 2) having a known history of mental illness; or 3) having a current diagnosis of mental illness; or 4) in need of mental health services.

Although a statewide study estimated that 50 percent of Pennsylvania's RCF population was mentally ill [3], the lower proportion identified here (27%) reflects the exclusion of persons the providers believed were too confused or agitated to complete the interviews required by the study. Nearly 70 percent of those approached completed the interview, yielding 195 baseline interviews. Non-respondents included 16 percent who were ineligible due to either physical illness or impaired cognitive function, and 14 percent refused to participate.

At Time 2, 142 residents (E = 69%; C = 76%) were available for interviews at their original facility (131 persons) or in an RCF to which they had been transferred (11 persons). Of these, 126 residents successfully completed the questionnaire, but staff interviews were obtained for all 142 residents. There were no significant differences between the treatment groups in their residential status at Time 2.

The Participating Facilities

Most experimental group residents (47%) lived in one large facility, a converted apartment block, and another 25 percent lived in another large home on the outskirts of town. The remaining 28 percent lived in four small facilities, three of which were owned and run cooperatively by a family group, and the fourth was owned and operated independently by a relative of that same family.

The milieu within these facilities lend insight into the intervention's lack of impact. Although PCH operators were cooperative with the workers, life in the homes went on without reference to the program. In the large urban facility, the 107 residents (half of whom were elderly) were periodically upset by extremely negative events. These incidents included allegations of thefts from residents, the rape and assault of a resident, and other events reminiscent of those that were alleged to have occurred in mental hospitals. This facility was the property of an absentee landlord who owned other "institutions," businesses, and offices in the county. A full-time administrator and staff worked hard assisting residents with medications, attending to their daily upkeep, and dealing with a variety of ongoing problems common to large agglomerations of troubled people. There were also ongoing staff issues including turnover, allegations of staff substance abuse, and improper handling of residents' behavior problems and substance abuse.

The second large facility housed sixty-three residents. Not as large as the other, it also had a full-time administrator, staff, and an absentee owner. This facility was somewhat less "troubled" than the first, perhaps because it was more rurally situated, and almost all of its residents were over the age of sixty. Although rare, there were upsetting events here as well. Generally the atmosphere was one of maintenance—where staff time was consumed by routine administrative tasks, residents physically or mentally decompensating, reports of resident misbehavior while in town, and the ongoing problem of finding competent personnel.

The three smaller facilities had a less disturbing atmosphere but were located in a very poor area of town at the center of its drug trade. The fourth small facility specialized in younger, more troubled ex-mental hospital patients and was frequently dealing with issues of resident misbehavior in the community. Although the resident composition was generally stable among these small homes, there was the problem of residents disappearing and later being found some place far away. The owners of these facilities frequently complained about trouble managing within the payment rates they received from their residents, all of whom were receiving SSI. As in the large facilities, these owners cooperated with the workers, but the routine of the facility went on parallel to the program workers' efforts.

The environment of the comparison group facilities mirrored that of the experimental group homes (both small and large), with administrators echoing the complaints regarding payment rates, staffing shortages, and chronic crises. The resident mix was also similar.

The twenty facilities within this study are obviously not representative of the universe of RCFs, however, based on interviews with state licensing officials and on our visits to numerous homes that were not included in this study, we believe that these residences are not atypical in size, ambiance, and composition of residents and staff. Although these facilities fall far below the lifestyle of a relatively small (but growing) proportion of RCFs catering to the wealthy and middle class, they are considerably better than a large number of unlicensed facilities or homes that are licensed but unwilling to be subject to public view. In these marginal facilities, resident life is even more stressed.

Measurement Variables

Baseline interviews were conducted between April and June, 1988, and the second data collection occurred one year later. Sample characteristics and intervention impact were measured by standardized instruments comprised of psychological scales with proven validity and other questions designed and pretested for this study. Separate interview schedules were used with residents and with staff members.

The resident questionnaire was adapted from the National Long Term Care Demonstration Baseline Assessment Instrument [15]. The interview covered demographic and medical information, the PGC Instrumental Activities of Daily Living Scale [16], the Short Portable Mental Status Questionnaire (SPMSQ) [17], and the Brief Symptom Inventory (BSI) [18]. The BSI, consisting of fifty-three five-point self-report Likert scales, measures the degree to which residents experience symptoms of various psychiatric disorders and yields nine separate symptom scores and a global score. Residents were also asked about their contact with friends and family, their perception of the RCF's home-likeness, and their ability to participate in activities.

The staff interview gathered supplementary information about the resident and ratings of resident disability. Some questions were parallel to those asked of the resident and were used as a measure of reliability. The questionnaire consisted of items from the National Long Term Care Demonstration staff interview, the Multidimensional Observation Scale for Elderly Subjects (MOSES) [19]— staff assessments of residents' functional ability and psychiatric symptomatology and residents' use of prescription medications and services respectively. Services measured were the amount of emergency and routine care received and the number of programs attended. Resident participation in activities was also considered.

Methods of Analyses

Characteristics of the experimental and comparison groups at baseline was accomplished by measures of central tendency and two-tailed t-tests for independent groups. Because differences (described below) were found in the age and gender distribution between the groups, they were further compared using analyses of covariance with the influence of these variables and group membership considered separately.

For posttest comparisons, a change score was computed for each measure reflecting mean differences between Time 1 and Time 2. An ANOVA then determined if one group changed significantly more than the other. To more clearly isolate the intervention impact, a series of regression analyses controlled for dissimilarities between the groups at baseline. Additional regression analyses were also conducted which included all possible interaction terms between the baseline score, age, gender, and group assignment.

RESULTS

Table 1 presents the demographic characteristics of the sample and reveals that the experimental and comparison groups were significantly different from one another on some key variables. Specifically, the comparison group was older, had more women, and fewer of its members entered the facility directly from a state mental hospital and more from another non-private dwelling.

Comparing Experimental and Comparison Groups on Dependent Variables (Table 2, Parts 1 and 2)

When initial dissimilarities were not controlled, the experimental group was healthier in cognitive functioning (as measured by the SPMSQ), ADL performance, on four of the BSI measures (interpersonal difficulties, depression, anxiety, and phobia), and in the general symptom inventory. Even after controlling for initial differences, the experimental group remained less impaired in ADL ability and were healthier on the BSI measures than the comparison group.

Table 1. Demographic Characteristics of Experimental Comparison and Total Groups

Variable	Experimental Group Baseline Value	Control Group Baseline Value	Total Group Baseline Value
Age (Mean)**	65.70[a]	69.90[a]	68.20[a]
Gender (%)**			
Male	62.00	38.00	47.70
Female	38.00	62.00	52.30
Race (%)			
White	65.70	55.20	62.60
Black/Other	34.30	44.80	37.40
Marital Status (%)			
Married	9.20	5.90	7.20
Widowed	31.60	29.70	30.40
Divorced	17.10	15.30	16.00
Separated	9.20	5.90	17.20
Never Married	32.90	43.20	39.20
Prior Residence (%)*			
Mental hospital	15.50	4.30	9.80
Non-private	8.50	18.30	14.50
Alone or family	58.00	63.00	61.10
Other RCF	17.00	14.00	14.50

*p < .05
**p < .01
[a]Standard Deviation of Age—E = 9.7; C = 9.6; T = 9.8

Several differences emerged as a result of age or gender. In the combined group, age was significantly related to intellectual impairment as measured by both the SPMSQ ($p < .001$) and the Moses Disorientation Scale ($p < .001$). Younger residents (50-70 years of age) had better self-care skills, participated in significantly more programs away from the facility, and received significantly more services from professionals than did their elder (71+ years of age) counterparts. There were no gender differences in these areas.

Staff also reported differences in psychotic symptoms related to age and gender. Females were described as more depressed ($p < .001$) and more irritable than males, and older residents as more withdrawn than younger ones.

Resident Characteristics

Surprisingly, staff and residents reported a remarkable lack of physical limitation. Perhaps reflecting sampling procedures, there was also little evidence of cognitive impairment and active psychiatric symptoms. The group average on the SPMSQ was 5.8, demonstrating only moderate intellectual impairment according to published norms [17]. On the Moses, over half (52.5%) of the residents were rated by staff as fully oriented.

Psychiatrically, residents reported few symptoms. On eight of the nine dimensional BSI measures, the means of the entire sample fell between the mean scores of normal non-patients and psychiatric outpatients [18]. Consistent with residents, staff reported low levels of all psychotic symptoms on the Moses scales.

Table 2 (Part 1) also shows that there is an uneven receipt of services and programs among residents. For example, nearly 16 percent received no routine professional services in a two-month period, 46 percent received four or fewer such services, while 38.3 percent received at least five professional services within the same time frame. Nearly half (47.9%) of all residents participated in no outside programs during a two-week period, over one-quarter attended between one and six programs, while 27 percent were in seven or more programs! These discrepancies were seen in both treatment groups.

Apparently, the core of this sample's disability was social marginality rather than physical impairment or overt psychiatric symptoms. Their major dysfunction was their inability to deal with the physical and social aspects of the larger world. For example, while 80 percent of the residents were able to manage basic activities of daily living, their difficulties dramatically increased when they needed to interact with others or to navigate the outside world. Nearly thirty-five percent of the residents reported that they were unable to buy things even when they had money; 52 percent were unable to use public transportation; and nearly 41 percent felt that they were unable to do things with other people! In contrast, only 16 percent reported an inability to clean their rooms.

Evidence of social marginality was also demonstrated by the 39 percent who never married and by the 25 percent who had nowhere to go when discharged

Table 2. Baseline and Change Scores of Experimental,
Comparison and Total Groups (Part 1)

	Experimental Group		Comparison Group		Total Group	
	Baseline	Time 2	Baseline	Time 2	Baseline	Time 2
Self Rated Health (%)						
Excellent/Good	67.10	59.60	54.70	60.80	60.00	60.30
Fair/Poor	32.90	40.40	45.30	39.20	40.00	39.70
Service Use (%) (2 mons)						
0 Routine svcs	9.10	5.70	19.80	19.10	15.50	14.10
1-4 Routine svcs	45.50	56.60	46.60	61.80	46.20	59.90
5+ Routine svcs	45.50	37.70	33.60	19.10	38.30	26.10
Number of Programs (%) (2 wks)						
0 Outside	49.40	56.60	47.00	48.30	47.90	51.40
1-6 Outside	27.30	37.70	23.90	18.00	25.30	25.40
7+ Outside	23.40	5.70	29.10	33.70	26.80	23.20
IADL/Social Ability (%)						
Do with others						
very much	30.10	19.60	30.70	34.60	30.50	29.00
somewhat	26.00	34.80	30.70	28.20	28.90	30.60
very little	43.90	45.70	38.60	37.20	40.60	40.30
Use public transportation						
very much	32.90	31.80	30.00	21.10	33.70	25.00
somewhat	16.20	18.20	13.60	18.40	14.70	18.30
very little	44.60	50.00	56.40	60.50	51.60	56.70
Buy at a store						
very much	45.40	44.20	37.70	44.00	40.90	36.40
somewhat	23.40	18.60	25.40	20.00	24.60	19.50
very little	31.20	37.20	36.80	36.00	34.60	36.40
Clean own room						
very much	65.80	67.40	66.10	51.90	66.00	57.60
somewhat	14.50	13.00	19.10	15.20	17.30	14.40
very little	19.70	19.60	14.80	32.90	16.40	28.00

Table 2. Baseline and Change Scores of Experimental Comparison and Total Groups (Part 2)

| | Experimental Group | | | | Comparison Group | | | | Total Group | | | |
| | Baseline | | Change | | Baseline | | Change | | Baseline | | Change | |
Variable	Mean	S.D.	Mean	S.D.	Mean	S.D.	Mean	S.D.	Mean	S.D.	Mean	S.D.
Chronic physical ills[a]	1.80	1.60	0.02	1.39	1.80	1.60	0.14	1.39	1.70	1.60	0.09	1.40
Orientation												
SPMSQ score	6.30	2.30	0.53	2.15	5.4**	2.20	−0.15	1.85	5.80	2.30	0.11	1.99
Moses score[a]	9.70	3.50	0.04	2.46	10.50	3.80	0.25	4.00	10.20	3.70	0.17	3.49
Self-Care (ADL) Ability												
Moses score[a]	7.40	1.80	0.47	2.02	8.6**	3.20	0.17	2.25	8.10	2.80	−0.07	2.19

*p < .05
**p < .01
[a]Higher scores = more disability; a positive change score denotes improvement.

211

from a mental hospital. Although 71 percent of the residents reported having relatives within twenty-five miles of the facility, there was little personal contact with them. Given their high level of physical functioning, it is likely that the residents' mental health histories impeded familial contact. These indications of social marginality were equally present in both the experimental and the comparison groups.

Thus, despite their relatively good physical health and lack of active psychotic symptoms, social marginality made the bulk of these residents sufficiently inappropriate that they were considered unacceptable at a senior center or at other community places. They appeared mentally disconnected and were awkward in handling social situations. The residents were often poorly groomed and may have been wearing dirty clothes or even clothes soiled by incontinence. Perhaps because they had no place to go, they tended to just hang around. In one instance, residents who left their facility for the day were asked not to "hang out" at a local fast food store. Unfortunately, individuals with these characteristics generally fall beneath the threshold of problems that mental health services are traditionally able to address.

Analysis of Intervention Impact

For the combined group, mean scores on psychological, functional, and medical scales remained stable in the year between the two data collections. A paired t-test revealed that in all but two instances, mean differences were not of sufficient magnitude to be statistically significant. The two variables that did have significant changes were perceived ability to perform IADLs ($p < .005$) and number of programs attended ($p < .01$). However, while the total sample significantly declined in these two areas, ANOVA testing showed neither group declined significantly more than the other.

In predicting Time 2 scores via stepwise regression, only the baseline score consistently entered into the equation. In virtually no instance was group membership a significant variable. There was only one measure (perceived ADL ability) on which a measure in addition to the baseline score was a significant predictor of Time 2. In this case, as age increased, residents' perceived ability to perform ADLs declined.

DISCUSSION

This section discusses three issues: 1) the poor response of counties and homes to participation in the study; 2) the lack of change in both the experimental and comparison groups; and 3) the implications for future programs and research.

Response to Participation in the Study

Statewide, out of sixty-two counties with RCFs, only two accepted the state funds to provide mental health services to RCF residents. At several meetings reluctance was expressed both to accept funds that the counties considered insufficient and to engage the problem of providing mental health services to RCF residents. For many, the grant was perceived as an attempt to co-opt them into taking responsibility for a problem that actually belonged to the state. For its part, the state Office of Mental Health felt that because so many of the residents of RCFs were elderly, the responsibility was with the state Department of Aging. That department replied that it had neither the budget nor responsibility to offer services to the mentally ill.

In Delaware County, the Office of Human Services was historically committed to dealing with the problems of ex-mental hospital patients, but it saw the younger ones as those who might "act out" and who, therefore, needed support. They ultimately agreed to focus on the more elderly resident but only if the investigators would lower the age range to be fifty years of age and over (rather than the original minimum of 60).

Among RCFs, reluctance to participate in the study, it was explained, stemmed from concerns that being identified as treating the mentally ill might label their residents negatively, discourage referrals, and possibly make the homes responsible for services they were not being funded to provide. As previously discussed, resistance to participation was evident on both ends of the RCF spectrum. The more exclusive facilities had a propensity to deny that mental illness was a problem for their residents, and that the "isolated few" were served by preexisting programs. Conversely, the more marginal facilities were reluctant to submit themselves to the scrutiny of a program worker or interviewer.

Although caution must be exercised in applying the present data to all RCFs, the twenty facilities that did participate are representative of the largest segment of the RCF world. This segment includes RCFs of all sizes, which serve poor and lower income residents without family to help care for them. Although many of these facilities are eager to capture a larger share of a more affluent market to offset low SSI rates, they are often unable to attract this resident due to marginal neighborhoods, rundown buildings, and threadbare (although clean) interiors. Already, greater numbers of affluent elderly people are seeking care in RCFs; when this demand is more clearly felt throughout the industry, the homes described here may indeed become the exception. However, at present, they represent the "norm."

The turf battle among units of government, the sense that mental health problems in boarding homes do not affect older residents, and the fear that acknowledging mental illness in boarding home clients will negatively impact business are tragic when their toll on residents is considered. In fact, most RCF residents are old and many of them are mentally ill and suffering from

Alzheimer's Disease. Residents who are not served have real needs that are not neatly separable into distinct mental health and aging domains. The result of sidestepping the true characteristics of RCF residents is that their needs are not addressed at all or only when they become severe. Programmatically, the sidestep means that scarce resources that might and that ought to be coordinated are dissipated by avoidance activity.

Impact of the Program

The workers responsible for providing services to the RCF residents were committed to a program that offered a combination of "on site" individual and group meetings, psychosocial rehabilitation sessions off site, and for some residents, participation at a senior center. Positive changes that have been noted anecdotally by caseworkers and facility staff include, for example, caseworkers' ability to obtain funding for prostheses, increases in the number of residents accepted into senior centers, and helping residents to secure funds withheld by relatives. Another encouraging note is that one of the participating agencies has recently planned and budgeted for a mental health clinic specifically responding to the special needs of geriatric mentally ill residents and reimbursable with medicaid funds.

Yet, the follow-up data do not demonstrate a significant impact in regard to the hypothesized outcomes. The remaining data collection, eighteen months after initiation of services, is still being analyzed, but it also shows little intervention impact. This lack of impact probably results from the residents' stability at baseline in most of the behaviors measured, from residents having different pathology than expected, and from an inadequately intense and structured intervention.

The final sample included 27 percent of the residents within the participating facilities—a rather substantial proportion. The program targeted people who were "mentally ill" but also "testable and likely to be cooperative." By intent, the program included not only elderly residents, but middle-aged ones as well. Thus, this sample under-represented the proportion of residents reported in a statewide survey [3] as demented (21.4%), very old (34%), and female (68.6%) and overrepresented men, the middle aged, and the young-old. Having excluded the most confused and symptomatic residents (the people for whom the instruments were intended), the resulting sample's scores were so near the top of the scales on the measures used that ceiling effects were likely to mask any evidence of improvement.

Furthermore, not all residents remained stable and in the facility. The retest sample includes only the subset of residents who were still in the RCF at Time 2—the group that is likely to have been the healthiest to begin with. We are currently analyzing our data to examine the baseline characteristics that may be predictive of those who died, were untestable, or moved to other levels of care.

Was wrong or inadequate treatment given? All four workers often had to work hard to get residents to participate in programs that were more demanding than they could easily manage. Thus, the workers had to constantly balance the conflicting priorities of their own judgment of the clients' needs, those of other systems (such as mental health and aging), and the abilities, interests, and priorities of the residents themselves. The result was less program delivery than we or the workers hoped.

Suggestions for Better Programming

The problems of marginally adjusted people are not easily addressed. By "marginal" we mean a person with a weak or immature ego who is unable to address the more complex demands of life. This inability may not be lack of intelligence but rather a timorousness or awkwardness in managing life's usual instrumental and interpersonal demands. These persons, while asymptomatic in the extreme psychotic sense, are inadequate for unsupported living. They may respond better if a much more structured program were offered to them. Gottesman argued in describing milieu treatment, that programs that are tightly structured to create demands like those in the "real" world, but at the margin of what the resident can manage, tend to stretch the ego and encourage its growth [20]. This theory is very similar to that of Carling and his co-workers [10, 11] when they describe, in situ treatment of ex-mental hospital patients.

An alternative approach to this sort of population is demonstrated in programs for the developmentally disabled, a number of which have been structured around the needs of people who are unlikely to reach significantly greater levels of performance. What those residents can do is meet the considerable demands of more or less independent structured living. Given this increased structure, they do remarkably well.

These intervention programs have successfully addressed several types of disabled clients, spanning the range between the independent community dwelling mentally ill and those with substantial and irreversible cognitive disability. Therefore, it seems likely that the generalized approach to building ego skills that these programs share will also be applicable to the broad spectrum of RCF residents.

The typical RCF is not funded to provide programs approaching the intensity and structure of the facilities just described. They see to it that the residents take medication, and that they are fed and clean. Providers often feel that to expect more engagement of the resident would either open the home up to charges of abusing the residents (if the engagement involved performing duties in the facility) or else require a level of staffing for which they are not paid. A move toward more appropriate programs would require differences in payment as well as in expectation of the role of the RCF as a "treatment" site. This study has clearly demonstrated that as they are now supported, the current environment within RCFs, particularly those serving poor, elderly, and mentally ill residents is not an effective treatment locale. Enhanced expectations and support for the facilities themselves can transform these residences into positive and safe environments in which marginal people may greatly enhance their capacity to interact with the world.

REFERENCES

1. National Association of Residential Care Facilities, *1987 Directory of Residential Care Facilities,* Richmond, Virginia, 1987.
2. N. D. Dittmar, G. P. Smith, J. C. Bell, C. B. C. Jones, and D. L. Manzanares, *Board and Care for Elderly and Mentally Disabled Populations: Volumes I-IV,* University of Denver, Denver Research Institute, Denver, 1983.
3. Conservation Company, *A Study of the Characteristics and Condition of Personal Care Home Residents in Pennsylvania—Volumes 1 & II,* Prepared for the Pennsylvania Departments of Public Welfare, Health, and Aging, Pennsylvania, 1988.
4. Office of Mental Health, *Mental Health Bulletin: Characteristics of Personal Care Home Residents in Pennsylvania,* Commonwealth of Pennsylvania, Department of Public Welfare, Harrisburg, Pennsylvania, November 1985.
5. L. E. Faulk, Jr., Quality of Life Factors in Board and Care Homes for the Elderly: A Hierarchical Model, *Adult Foster Care Journal,* 2:2, pp. 100-117, 1988.
6. S. Sherwood and L. Gruenberg, *Domiciliary Care Management Information System* (mimeo), Hebrew Home for the Aged, Department of Social Gerontological Research, Boston, 1979.
7. R. J. Newcomer and L. Grant, *Residential Care Facilities: Understanding Their Role and Improving Their Effectiveness,* (Policy Paper No. 2 [1]), Institute for Health and Aging, University of California at San Francisco, San Francisco, 1981.
8. R. Stone and R. J. Newcomer, The State Role in Board and Care Housing, in *Long Term Care of the Elderly: Public Policy Issues,* C. Harrington, et al. (eds.), Sage Publications, Beverly Hills, California, pp. 177-197, 1985.
9. L. Gottesman and E. M. Brody, Psychological Intervention Programs Within the Institutional Setting, in *Long-term Care: A Handbook for Researchers, Planners, and Providers,* S. Sherwood (ed.), Spectrum Publications, New York, pp. 455-509, 1975.
10. A. K. Blanch, P. J. Carling, and R. Ridgway, Normal Housing with Specialized Supports: A Psychiatric Rehabilitation Approach to Living in the Community, *Rehabilitation Psychology, 33*:1, pp. 47-55, 1988.
11. G. Fairweather (ed.), The Fairweather Lodge: A Twenty-five Year Perspective, in *New Directions in Mental Health Services,* No. 7, Jossey-Bass, San Francisco, 1980.
12. F. Lawrence and P. J. Volland, The Community Care Program: Description and Administration, *Adult Foster Care Journal,* 2:1, pp. 26-37, 1988.
13. J. S. Oktay, K. Horwitz, and P. J. Volland, Evaluation of the Quality of Care and the Cost of the Community Care Program, *Adult Foster Care Journal,* 2:1, pp. 52-71, 1988.
14. P. J. Volland, Foster Care for the Frail Elderly, *Adult Foster Care Journal,* 2:1, pp. 72-82, 1988.

15. B. R. Phillips, S. A. Stephens, J. J. Cerf, et al. *The Evaluation of the National Long Term Care Demonstration: Survey Data Collection Design and Procedures,* Mathematica Policy Research, Princeton, New Jersey, 1986.

16. M. P. Lawton, Assessing the Competence of Older People, in *Research Planning & Action for the Elderly,* D. Kent, R. Kastenbaum, and S. Sherwood (eds.), Behavioral Publications, New York, pp. 122-143, 1972.

17. Duke University Center for the Study of Aging and Human Development, *Multidimensional Functional Assessment: The OARS Methodology,* Duke University, Durham, North Carolina, 1978.

18. L. R. Derogatis and P. M. Spencer, *The Brief Symptom Inventory (BSI) Administration, Scoring & Procedures Manual—I,* Clinical Psychometrics Research, Baltimore, 1982.

19. E. Helmes, K. G. Csapo, and J. A. Short, *A Survey of Psychological Functioning in the Institutionalized Elderly in Ontario,* Bulletin #8605 ISBN #0711-0612, The University of Western Ontario, Department of Psychiatry, London, Ontario, 1987.

20. L. Gottesman, Milieu Treatment of the Aged in Institutions, *The Gerontologist, 13*:1, pp. 23-26, 1973.

Contributors

LOURDES BIRBA, M.S.G., Southern California Edison Company, Rosemead, California.

JENNIFER DAVIS-BERMAN is an Associate Professor in the Department of Sociology, Anthropology and Social Work at the University of Dayton. She is currently exploring the impact of experiential-based groups on depressive symptoms and self-efficacy in older adults. She also teaches courses on Aging and Death and Dying at the university. Finally, she is involved in a counseling practice specializing in providing mental health services to older adults.

SALLY R. ESSER, M.D., St. Mary's Hospital Family Practice, Milwaukee, Wisconsin.

JAMES F. FRIES, M.D. is Professor of Medicine at Stanford University School of Medicine. He received his A.B. from Stanford in 1960, his M.D. from Johns Hopkins in 1964. He trained at Hopkins and Stanford, and was board certified in internal medicine in 1968 and rheumatology in 1970. He has been on the Stanford Faculty since 1970. He has been Carnegie-Commonwealth Clinical Scholar, an Arthritis Foundation Clinical Scholar, and a Fellow at the Center for Advanced Study in Behavioral Sciences. He has published over 180 scientific articles and eleven books and is on multiple review and editorial boards.

His research activities have centered around the long-term outcomes of chronic diseases and the aging process and the factors which are associated, utilizing large computer data banks. He introduced the time-oriented medical record and systematic outcome assessment with the Health Assessment Questionnaire (HAQ). He is Director of the National Arthritis Data Resource (ARAMIS), a large AIDS data bank (ATHOS), a Post-marketing Drug Surveillance Program (PORTHOS), and is Associate Director of the Stanford Arthritis Center (SAC).

In 1980 he presented the landmark paradigm of The Compression of Morbidity, establishing the underlying theoretical structures and goals of health promotion as improvement of life quantity in an era where future increases in longevity would be less, and has since been exploring the policy implications and opportunities of this paradigm. In 1984 he developed the Healthtrac health promotion and disease prevention program, with an emphasis upon health improvement, medical cost reduction, and rigorous proof of effectiveness; Healthtrac is now the leading and best-documented program in the country, with well over a million participants. He is Chairman of The Healthtrac Foundation, which annually awards the Healthtrac Prize to that individual judged to have had the greatest impact upon improving the health of the public.

LEONARD E. GOTTESMAN, PH.D. has been the principal and an active participant in a number of projects dedicated to developing and evaluating innovative services which help to keep people independent, self-sufficient, and satisfied with their lives. He has assisted the U.S. Department of Health and Human Services, AoA, NIMH, the Health Care Financing Administration and the states of Pennsylvania, Maryland, Maine, Delaware, Massachusetts, Texas, New York, West Virginia, and Ohio to develop both health and social services to help dependent and disabled persons to remain independent.

Dr. Gottesman received his Ph.D. in Psychology from the University of Chicago in 1959. He has served as Professor of Psychology at the University of Michigan, Director of Technical Assistance at the Philadelphia Geriatric Center, and on the faculty of Temple University, Villanova University's Human Organization Services Program. He is currently on the faculty of the West Chester University Psychology Department where he teaches course in Organizational Psychology, Personality Theory and Human Development. His areas of specialization are program evaluation, organizational change, and human development.

JOCELYN HAMEL, M.A., Lakehead University, Thunder Bay, Ontario.

JON HENDRICKS, PH.D, is Professor and Chair, Department of Sociology, Oregon State University. He is President, Association for Gerontology in Higher Education and has previoulsy served as an officer of The Gerontological Society of America and The American Sociological Association. Hendricks is Associate Editor for the *International Journal of Aging and Human Development*, Series Editor for *Perspectives on Aging and Human Development Series*, and Consulting Editor for Gerontology, Baywood Publishing Company, Inc., NY. Hendricks is a member of Worldwide Umbrella Exchange and is widely published in the field of social gerontology.

PATRICIA A. HILL, M.A. currently works in Regional Health Promotion Planning in Nelson, British Columbia, Canada.

SAMUEL HIMMELFARB, Department of Psychology and Urban Studies Center, University of Louisville, Louisville, Kentucky.

HOWARD B. KAPLAN, PH.D. is Distinguished Professor of Sociology, Mary Thomas Marshall Professor of Liberal Arts, and Director of the Laboratory for Studies of Social Deviance at Texas A&M University. He received his Ph.D. in Sociology from New York University in 1958. During his career he has been awarded a Russell Sage Post-doctoral Fellowship, a Milbank Memorial Fund Faculty Fellowship, and currently holds a Research Scientist Award from the National Institute on Drug Abuse. He has served as editor of the *Journal of Health and Social Behavior* (1979-1981) and as chairman of the Drug Abuse Epidemiology and Prevention Research Review Committee of the National Institute on Drug Abuse (1985-1990). His research focuses on testing theoretically informed models of social-psychological antecedents and consequences of deviant adaptations to stress using a panel of 9,000 subjects tested up to five times between adolescence (junior high school) and young adulthood (the third decade of life). This work and related research reentered the field to follow the cohort into the fourth decade of life and to test the children of the cohort who have reached the same age that their parents were when they were first interviewed as junior high school students. He has 135 publications including seven books and ninety peer-reviewed articles appearing in such outlets as *American Journal of Sociology, Journal of Health and Social Behavior, Social Psychology Quarterly, Social Forces, American*

Journal of Psychiatry, Archives of General Psychiatry, and numerous other sociological, psychiatric, and interdisciplinary behavioral science journals.

KATHLEEN KENNEDY, PH.D. is currently the Director of Public Health Programs for Mercy Health Plan, a Medicaid-managed care organization. She is responsible for the planning, implementation, and evaluation of outreach and case-management programs which address the public and personal health needs of members. Dr. Kennedy's previous professional experiences include community health nursing and adolescent counseling.

Dr. Kennedy received her Ph.D. in Health Education at Temple University. She has served on the faculty of Widener University. Dr. Kennedy's areas of public health specialization are behavioral health and infectious diseases.

JOHN A. KROUT, PH. D., is Professor of Health Sciences and Director, Gerontology Institute of Ithaca College. He previously was Professor of Sociology and Director of the Health Care Administration program and coordinator of the gerontology concentration at the State University of New York—College of Fredonia. He has published thirty articles in a wide range of academic journals and has made some seventy-five presentations at national and state conferences. He has received ten grants to support his research program on rural aging issues, which focuses on community-based services. His books include *The Aged in Rural America* and *Senior Centers in America* as well as several bibliographies on rural aging. He has conducted national studies on senior centers, Area Agencies on Aging, and case management for the rural elderly, with the majority of his funding coming from the AARP Andrus Foundation. He currently serves as a consultant to the National Institute on Multipurpose Senior Centers and Community Focal Points and recently spent three years as a project specialist for the National Resource Center for the Rural Elderly. He has served as a member of the delegate council of the National Council on the Aging's National Center on Rural Aging. He currently serves on the boards of directors of several state and local aging organizations and on the editorial boards of *The Gerontologist* and the *Journal of Applied Gerontology,* and is Fellow of the Gerontological Society of America.

KAREN S. KUBENA, PH.D., is Associate Professor of Nutrition and of Food Science and Technology, Texas A&M University. Completing degrees at the University of Wisconsin-Madison, Mississippi State University, and Texas A&M University, she began as Assistant Professor at Texas A&M in 1982 and now serves as Section Leader for the Human Nutrition Section, Administrator for the Combined Graduate Degree-Dietetic Internship and Director, Didactic Program in Dietetics. As a registered and licensed dietitian, her experience includes a number of years as a dietetic practitioner and department head in health care facilities. The relationship between diet and health has been the focus of her research. Metabolism of minerals, especially magnesium, and fat has been investigated in laboratory animals and humans. Human studies have targeted interactions among dietary intake, nutritional status, health and other factors, such as health behaviors and social support. Populations investigated include elderly individuals, adolescents, and pregnant women. She has authored or co-authored more than fifty papers and abstracts in refereed journals. Responsibilities also include teaching courses in nutrition in the life cycle and nutrition in disease. Dr. Kubena is a member of the American Institute of Nutrition, American Society of Clinical Nutrition, Institute of Food Technologists and the

American Dietetic Association. She has held offices at the national level in the American Dietetic Association and in the Faculty of Nutrition at Texas A&M.

WENDALL A. LANDMANN, Ph.D., Professor Emeritus, retired in the late 1980s after a career in which he was recognized as an authority on protein metabolism. After completing degrees at the University of Illinois and Purdue University, his first area of research was meat science, in conjunction with which he held positions at the Argonne National Laboratory in Lemont, Illinois, and the American Meat Institute Foundation, Chicago. In 1964, he joined the faculty of Texas A&M University as Professor of Biochemistry and Biophysics and of Animal Science. During the 1970s, he served as Head, Department of Biochemistry and Biophysics. It was at this time that he became interested in nutrition which was reflected in a new research direction of protein metabolism in humans. After returning to a faculty position in 1979, Dr. Landmann taught and conducted research in human nutrition until his retirement. Over his career, he was active in professional and honor societies, including Sigma Xi and Phi Kappa Phi, often holding offices. He is deceased.

J. PAUL LEIGH received a Ph.D. in economics from the University of Wisconsin, Madison, in 1979. He is a professor of economics at San Jose State University and a senior research economist at the Stanford Medical Center. He has published over 100 scientific articles. His book, *Death within Occupations and Industries,* details causes of job-related deaths within over 250 jobs. It will be published by Greenwood in February 1995.

MICHAEL I. MacENTEE is a Professor in the Faculty of Dentistry and Chairman of the Division of Prosthodontics, Department of Clinical Dental Sciences, University of British Columbia.

WILLIAM ALEX McINTOSH has an M.S. and Ph.D. in Sociology from Iowa State University. He has taught since 1975 at Texas A&M University, where he holds a joint appointment in the Departments of Sociology and Rural Sociology and is a member of the Graduate Faculty of Nutrition. McIntosh is former President of the Association for the Study of Food in Society and former Book Review Editor for *Rural Sociology.* He is the current Book Review Editor for *Food and Foodways.* McIntosh has received research support from NIH, NIDA, USDA, the Texas Department of Human Resources.

Much of his research in the past decade has centered on the relationship between food and nutrition, on the one hand, and social relationships, on the other. He has investigated the impact of the elderly's social support network on their nutritional health and is currently examining the impact of family structure on adolescent's development of nutritional risk factors of cardiovascular disease. He also is completing a manuscript for Plenum Press entitled *Sociologies of Food and Nutrition.* His work has appeared in the *American Journal of Sociology, Sociological Quarterly, Social Science Quarterly, Rural Sociology, The International Journal of Aging and Human Development, Journal of Aging and Health, and Appetite.*

JAY MEDDIN is Senior Lecturer in Health Sciences in the School of Public Health at Curtin University of Technology, Perth Western Australia.

He has a long-term interest in subjective well-being among the aged, and his current research deals with meaning or purpose in life for older persons.

DR. MICHÁL E. MOR-BARAK is an Associate Professor at the University of Southern California's School of Social Work and holds a joint appointment with the

Andrus Center's School of Gerontology. Prior to assuming an academic appointment, Dr. Mor-Barak had a number of positions working in welfare agencies and in industrial settings. In corporate settings, she has worked in clinical practice, program development, training and consultation positions. She was also involved in the evaluation of a state-wide case-management demonstration project for the elderly, and currently serves as a consultant to Southern California Edison on issues of health care provision to their retirees.

Dr. Mor-Barak teaches research, human behavior, social work practice in work settings, and a statistics course in the doctoral program. Her research interests are in industrial social work and gerontology, and she currently supervises (with Dr. Andrew Scharlach) the research effort evaluating corporate sponsored geriatric health clinics which employ a multi-disciplinary case-managed approach. Additionally, she is investigating the determinants of successful linkages between older job-seekers and employers.

Dr. Mor-Barak's publications are in the areas of industrial social work, gerontology, and crisis intervention, including a book entitled, *Social Networks and Health of the Frail Elderly*. She has made conference presentations on the relationship between social networks and the health of the elderly, and has given workshops on stress management and the employment of the elderly.

JANA MOSSEY, PH.D., is an Associate Professor in the Department of Medicine and Psychiatry at the Medical College of Pennsylvania. She holds a Ph.D. in Epidemiology from the University of North Carolina, and is also a masters prepared Clinical Nurse Specialist in psychiatry. Her research focuses on the relationships between psychosocial factors and well-being. She has studied the importance of self-rated health for mortality in older individuals and of elevated depressive symptoms for recovery from hip fracture. She is currently studying the costs of subdysthymic depressive symptoms as indicated by excess disability and excess use of health services.

STANLEY A. MURRELL, PH.D., is currently Professor of Psychology and Director of the Clinical Psychology Ph.D. Program at the University of Louisville. He has served on the editorial boards of *Psychology and Aging* and *Journal of Gerontology: Psychological Sciences*.

MARTHA A. NELSON has recently joined the Rural Sociology Department and the Texas State Data Center at Texas A&M University as a Research Assistant. She is responsible for conducting demographic research for the state. Martha received her M.S. in Sociology, with an emphasis in Gerontology, from Texas A&M University. Since graduating, she has worked as a Policy Analyst for the Texas Legislature and as a marketing and social science researcher for a research firm in Pennsylvania.

ELLEN PESKIN, M.A., is a Research Project Director at the Leonard Davis Institute of Health Economics at the University of Pennsylvania School of Medicine. She has conducted research in the fields of mental health and health care policy and program evaluation, pharmacoeconomics and psychometrics.

Ms. Peskin earned her degree at Temple University. She has been affiliated with the Community Services (Narberth, Pennsylvania), the National Board of Medical Examiners (Philadelphia, Pennsylvania), and the University of Pennsylvania.

JAMES F. PHIFER, Department of Psychology and Urban Studies Center, University of Louisville, Louisville, Kentucky.

KEN J. ROTENBERG received his Ph.D. in Developmental Psychology from the University of Western Ontario in London, Ontario. He is an Associate Professor in the Psychology Department at Lakehead University and is currently the Chair of the department. To date, Dr. Rotenberg has published two books and approximately fifty articles that reflect his interest in social development across the life span.

ANDREW E. SCHARLACH is an Associate Professor of Social Welfare at the University of California at Berkeley, where he holds the Eugene and Rose Kleiner Chair in Aging and directs the Gerontology specialization in the School of Social Welfare.

Dr. Scharlach has published extensively on the needs of older adults and their families, particularly with regard to employee elder care responsibilities and adults' reactions to parental death. He is a leading national expert in the area of employee dependent care, and he consults extensively regarding the development and evaluation of work and family programs. Dr. Scharlach's first book is entitled *Elder Care and the Work Force: Blueprint for Action.*

Dr. Scharlach received a B.A. in mathematics from the University of California at Berkeley, an M.S. in social service from Boston University, and a Ph.D. in psychology from Stanford University. He is a Diplomate in Clinical Social Work, a Fellow of the Gerontological Society of America, and is included in *Who's Who in California, Who's Who in the West, Who's Who of Emerging Leaders in America,* and *Who's Who in Gerontology.*

JACQUE SOKOLOV, M.D., Southern California Edison Company, Rosemead, California.

G. ELAINE STOLAR is Director of the School of Social Work at the University of British Columbia. He research and teaching focus on the psycho-social aspects of health and illness, and the process of aging.

HOWARD TURNER, MSW, is currently serving as an Adjunct Assistant Professor in Sociology at the University of Michigan—Flint. He is a Ph.D. Candidate in sociology at the University of Kentucky where he received a graduate certificate in gerontology. He is pursuing research in the area of older persons as volunteers for his doctoral studies. In addition to mental health issues in later life, Mr. Turner has published in the area of older volunteers and the area of health care decision-making in later life.

ALAN VAUX, Southern Illinois University.

PETER VITALIANO, Ph.D. Associate Professor, Department of Psychiatry and Behavioral Sciences, University of Washington.